RULES OF MEDICAL TERMINOLOGY

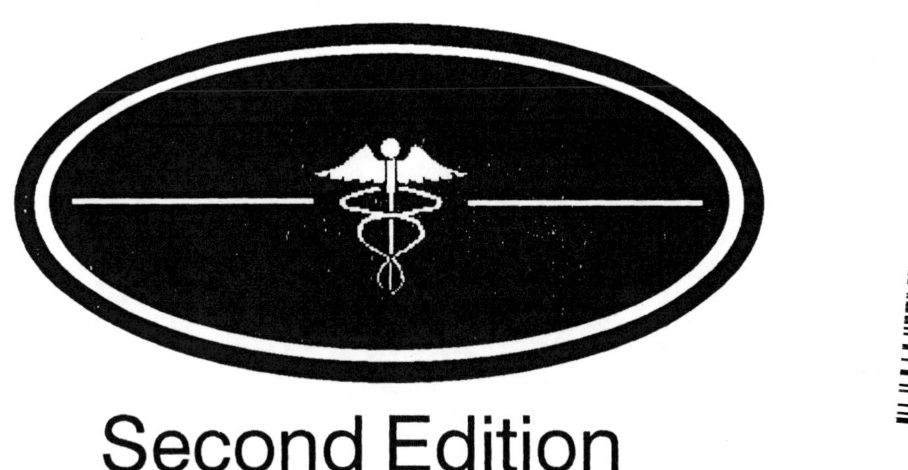

Second Edition

Lois Irby Mack, M.S., RN, CMA-C
Assistant Professor of Medical Assisting, Retired
Cuyahoga Community College, Metropolitan Campus
Cleveland, Ohio

KENDALL/HUNT PUBLISHING COMPANY
4050 Westmark Drive   Dubuque, Iowa 52002

Artwork by Beth Young.

CONTENTS

ACKNOWLEDGMENTS

To a great team:

Diane (Dede) Axthelm, Alice Kruse and Kathleen Malinkey, the eagle-eyes of scrutiny for the manuscript;

Dr. Theresa Offenberger and Charles T. Brown, fellow faculty members who were users of and made suggestions for this work;

and especially to:

Orene Anthony, a very brave lady who overcame great odds in her life and, by example, encouraged – badgered – me into completion of this work.

To each and the many others – other faculty, full- and part-time and students, I give my heartfelt thanks. Without you this would not exist.

PREFACE

Every generation, work specialty, and geographical group has a language of its own which is readily used and understood by its members. For instance, the word "nipple" has very different meanings when used by a mother – part of the breast or the mouth piece of the baby's nursing bottle, or by the plumber – a short piece of pipe with threads at both ends. A "chunk" is a substantial mass of something but in some parts of the country it means to throw. In each group it is of utmost importance that all persons within that group use and understand its own form of communication. Medical terminology is the language which is special to the medical field.

This book is designed as a very basic systematic method of structuring words of the language using its parts, components, to form properly spelled words. Most medical professionals learn the language of medicine as we learn our geographic or ethnic language – by hearing and speaking it. Reading or speaking does not always give precision to the understanding which is so necessary in a specialty. We frequently assume to understand meanings; not infrequently these assumptions are incomplete and/or incorrect.

This book does not consider dialect or pronunciation in the discussions and activity sections. We are a diverse society; pronunciation is an outgrowth of how and what we are taught. Our teachers are diverse in their native languages, educational backgrounds and learned pronunciation as were their teachers. It is becoming increasingly difficult to declare the correct pronunciation of some words but, more importantly, the spelling and meanings should remain constant.

INTRODUCTION

The goal of this book is to give the student the methods and tools which will enable them to read and spell terms used in the written and spoken language of medicine. This will be done by learning:

- the elements/components as they are used in the field of medicine;
- the rules of how to synthesize/word build correctly spelled terms;
- how to analyze medical terms in order to arrive at a reasonable definition.

This is a book of methodology and is not intended as a complete text of medical terminology, hence the inclusions of only those systems that best give the learner the broadest exposure to all the rules governing the structuring of medical terminology.

Because the instructor will be using some very common terms in explaining this language it is important to understand the meaning of these very basic words which we all assume we properly understand.

syllable   a sound within a word which usually has no meaning but by changing the syllables (sounds) within a word changes the word completely.

Both of these words have two syllables but one sound in each word has been changed to make a new word, e.g.:

WORD	SYLLABLES	
staple	sta	ple
people	peo	ple

word   is a unit of communication, written or spoken; it may not be divided into smaller units and retain its meaning, e.g.:

blood – the fluid of the circulatory system
pressure – the exertion of force

term   is a word or group of words that designate a specific something or specific concept. The group of words combine to convey a specific idea, e.g.:

blood pressure – the measurable pressure of the blood against the wall of an artery.

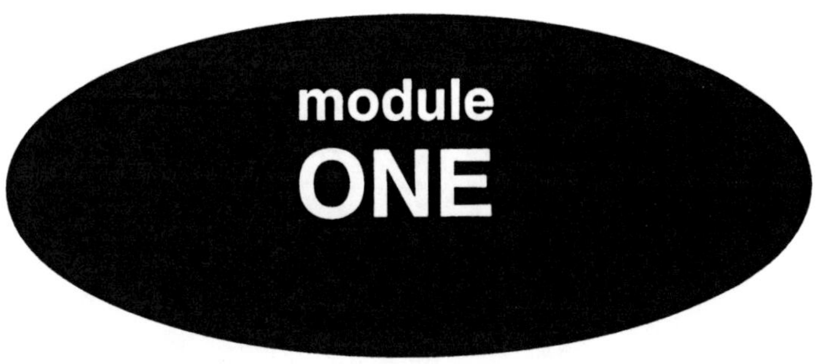

Vocabulary

Vocabulary

Selected terms:

1.	acute	of short duration, relatively severe, rapid onset
2.	acquired	occurring after birth, not hereditary
3.	anastomosis	a natural or surgical joining of two or more tubular structures or nerves for continuous flow and to form a communication
4.	anomaly	malformation, abnormal
5.	appendage	an attached part, e.g., arm, nose, breasts
6.	aspiration	to draw out of a cavity by suction
7.	atresia	absence of a normal body opening, either congenital or pathological
8.	autopsy	examination of a body after death
9.	benign	not malignant, generally not life threatening, good prognosis
10.	biopsy	microscopic examination of tissues excised during life to aid in making diagnosis
11.	cancer	general term for any malignant condition
12.	chronic	of long duration; continuous for long period of time
13.	congenital	born with; present at birth
14.	connective tissue	tissue which supports and connects other tissues or parts; does not include epithelial tissue
15.	diagnosis	to determine the nature of disease; an intellectual guess
16.	disease	any illness having a given set of clinical signs/symptoms and laboratory findings peculiar to it
17.	dissection	to cut apart, to separate tissues
18.	epithelial	tisssue which covers the body or organ in a continuous covering
19.	etiology	the study of the cause of disease
20.	excision	to cut out, complete cutting out
21.	extremity	an extreme part/end; distal end
22.	hernia	protrusion of a tissue or organ through a defect in muscle
23.	herniation	abnormal protrusion of all or part of an organ through a defect or normal opening in any tissue
24.	idiopathic	of unknown origin
25.	incision	to cut, cutting into

Selected terms:

26.	infection	presence of pathological organism activity in the body
27.	inflammation	reaction of body to trauma (heat, redness, swelling and pain and/or itching)
28.	kinesis	movement or motion of the body
29.	malignant	life threatening, cancerous growth; harmful to life
30.	metastasis	movement of harmful organism or body cells (esp. cancer cells) from one location in the body to another without direct connection
31.	mucosa	mucous membrane which lines all organs and cavities that connect to the outside; epithelial tissue (e.g., gingiva, lining of Alimentary Tract)
32.	mucus	fluid produced by the mucosa
33.	neoplasm	new and abnormal tissue; tumor
34.	paralysis	inability to move voluntarily – temporary or permanent
35.	parenchyma	functional tissue or structure
36.	prognosis	forecast of probable outcome
37.	prolapse	a falling down or dropping down of an organ or internal part
38.	resection	partial excision of a tissue or structure
39.	rupture	the abrupt separation of tissues
40.	serosa	tissue that lines all closed cavities of body (cranium, thorax, abdomen) and covers all organs within the cavity; also called serous membrane. Fluid of this tissue is serum or serous fluid
41.	signs	objective observations of bodily dysfunction (fever, cough, rash)
42.	sphincter	circular muscle controlling an orifice
43.	symptoms	subjective complaints of bodily dysfunction (cold, pain, headache)
44.	syndrome	combination of signs and/or symptoms that together constitute a distinct picture of an abnormal condition
45.	trauma	insult to body by injury or disease
46.	tumor	new overgrowth of tissue forming an abnormal mass; neoplasm
47.	viscera	internal organs enclosed within a cavity

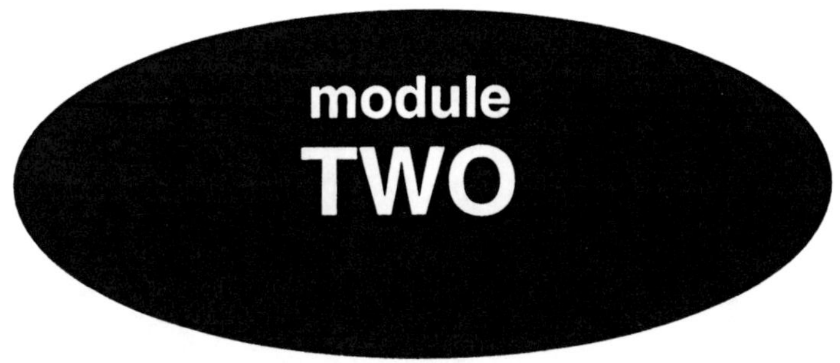

Elements of Word Formation

— Objectives —

Upon completion of this module the student should be able to:

1. Classify components by type: prefix, suffix, root stem or combining form, from a given list.

2. Demonstrate recognition of purpose and placement of each component by correctly building words from given component problems.

3. Correctly complete the activity portion of this module.

An understanding and knowledge of components and how they are used is necessary. A component is a part of a word that has a meaning of its own but may not be used as a word. Some, because of frequent usage in today's medical language are accepted as words; these are exceptions to the rules. There are four basic components:

1. The *Word Root*/Anatomic Root/Root Stem
2. The *Combining Form*/Root Word
3. The *Prefix*
4. The *Suffix*

For convenience of learning:

- All prefixes have a hyphen at the end of the component to indicate all other components follow.

- All suffixes have a hyphen at the beginning of the component to indicate all other components precede it. Never use a capital letter after the hyphen.

- All root words (combining forms or root stems) will have *NO* hyphen; their placement in a word depends on the other components used to form a word.

Definitions

A. Anatomic Root

A Word Root/Root Stem/Anatomic Root is the main body or basic core of a medical term. It usually refers to a human body organ or function and it is used like the noun of a sentence. The Root Stem will represent something that can be seen or felt — it appeals to the senses. Not all anatomic word roots will end with a consonant.

Examples of root stems are listed below.

Examples	*Meaning*
a. enter	intestine
b. col	colon, large intestine
c. stomat	mouth
d. dent	tooth/teeth

Examples	*Meaning*
e. gen	knee
f. chol	bile
*g. angi	vessel

*Not all anatomic roots end with a consonant.

Combining Vowels

A *Combining Vowel* is a vowel that is added to each word root to facilitate pronunciation and to allow the combining of other word roots and/or suffixes. The most frequently used combining vowel is "o." The presence or absence of the combining vowel *does not alter the meaning* of an anatomic root, however the combining vowel *does* alter spelling. The presence or absence of a combining vowel can cause a medical term to be misspelled.

Some anatomic roots end in a vowel, e.g. oste. The vowel is a part of the anatomic root; the addition of a combining vowel must be considered for this component to be combined with other components. Despite the presence of a vowel at the end of a word root there is still only one combining vowel.

B. Combining Form/Root Word

A *Combining Form*/Root Word is a component that results from combining an *anatomic root* with a *combining vowel*. In other words the anatomic root plus combining vowel equals a combining form.

EXAMPLE:

Word Root	+ *Combining Vowel*	= *Combining Form*	*Definition*
a. enter	o	entero	intestines
b. col	o	colo	colon
c. stomat	o	stomato	mouth
d. dent	o	dento	tooth/teeth
e. gen	u	genu	knee
f. chol	e	chole	bile
g. angi	o	angio	vessel

NOTE: The addition of the combining vowel to the word root/root stem does *not* change the meaning of the component.

Root Stem	*Combining Form*
gastr means stomach	gastro means stomach
oste means bone	osteo means bone

C. Prefix

A *Prefix* is a component attached to the *beginning* of a word to qualify its meaning. A prefix is a word beginning. The spelling of prefix does not change when placed before other components. The meaning of the word is not changed but is made more specific.

Examples		*Meaning*
a.	hemi-	half
b.	a-, an-	not, without
c.	auto-	self
d.	intra-	within, inside
e.	anti-	against
f.	di-	twice
g.	poly-	much, many
h.	hyper-	above, excessive
i.	hypo-	below, deficient
j.	sub-	under
k.	retro-	behind, backward
l.	trans-	across
m.	quadri-	four

D. Suffix

A *Suffix* is the component added to the end of a word to give it meaning. The spelling of a suffix does not change when added to other components. By changing the suffix the meaning of the word changes completely. Remember: because a suffix is attached at the end of other components, the first letter is NEVER capitalized. All words must have a suffix ending.

Examples		*Meaning*
a.	-osis	increase in condition, abnormal condition
b.	-tasis	stretching
c.	-itis	inflammation of
d.	-ectomy	excision
e.	-emesis	vomiting
f.	-penia	deficiency or decrease

Suffixes may be diagnostic, operative, symptomatic, an adjective or a noun.

1. **Diagnostic Suffixes** define or identify condition or disease.

Examples	*Meaning*
a. -ectasis	distention, dilation
b. -megalia	enlarged, large
c. -lithiasis	presence of stones in a structure of the body

2. **Operative Suffixes** describe or identify surgical or medical procedures.

Examples	*Meaning*
a. -ostomy	more or less permanent opening
b. -desis	surgical binding
c. -lithotomy	incision made for removal of stones from the body

3. **Symptomatic Suffixes** describe symptoms.

Examples	*Meaning*
a. -esthesia	feeling, sensation
b. -dipsia	thirst
c. -genic	originating in

4. **Noun Suffix** is a word or word root with an added noun ending, e.g., -ium, -ia, -es, -s, used at the end of a medical word in place of a suffix. Any anatomical part may be used as a noun suffix indicating a condition affecting that part. A noun suffix may be used as a word. A hyphen is used to indicate the word is being used as a noun suffix, otherwise it will be considered a word.

   When a word is used as a noun suffix, it joins the root stem with the combining vowel in place.

Examples	*Meaning*
a. -cervix (word used as suffix to indicate something present in that part)	condition affecting the neck
b. -glossia (-ia use indicates some type of abnormal condition)	condition affecting the tongue
c. -lith(s)	stone(s)

Common Noun Suffixes Composed of Word Root
Plus a Suffix

Noun Suffix	Meaning of Suffix	Root Stem Origin	Noun Ending
d. –algia	pain	alg	–ia
e. –cranium	(condition of) the skull	crani	–ium
f. –graphy	process of recording	graph	–y
g. –otomy	incision	tom	–y
h. –pathy	disease	path	–y
i. –phagia	swallow, eat, ingest	phag	–ia
j. –phonia	voice	phon	–ia
k. –plasty	surgical reconstruction	plast	–y

5. **Adjective Suffix** qualifies or modifies the word root.

   Examples   *Meaning*

   a. -al   pertaining to

   b. -ous   full of

   c. -ic   pertaining to

Student Practice Activities

Activity 1

Component Identification

Identify each of the following types of components.
Mark **S**-suffix; **P**-prefix; **CF**-combining form/root word; **A**-anatomic root/root stem/word root

1. -rrhage	S		11. col	A
2. -glossia	S		12. brady-	P
3. myo	CF		13. -pathy	S
4. arthr	A		14. dactylo	CF
5. -otomy	S		15. peri-	P
6. post-	P		16. stomat	A
7. gloss	A		17. -malacia	S
8. anti-	P		18. rachio	CF
9. hyper-	P		19. my	A
10. -itis	S		20. dent	A

Activity 2

Match A through F with their definitions (1-6).

A. anatomic root/root stem/word root   C. component   E. term

B. combining form/root word   D. syllable   F. word

1. Part of a word that has no meaning of its own; the sound(s) that make a word. _____________

2. A basic unit of written or oral communication.   _____________

Activity 2

(continued)

3. Part of a word that has a meaning of its own but cannot stand alone.   ___________

4. Main body or basic core of a medical term.   ___________

5. A word or group of words that implies a specific idea.   ___________

6. The anatomic root plus a vowel added to facilitate pronunciation and allow   ___________
   for the joining of more than one component.

Activity 3

Underline the combining vowel in each of the following:

1. gastro
2. viri
3. carpo
4. osteo
5. genu

6. chole
7. tracheo
8. chondro
9. angio
10. entero

Activity 4

Turn these components into combining forms if necessary.

1. gloss   ___________________________
2. colo   ___________________________
3. esophag   ___________________________
4. stomat   ___________________________
5. osteo   ___________________________

6. myelo   ___________________________
7. chondr   ___________________________
8. myos   ___________________________
9. angio   ___________________________
10. dento   ___________________________

Activity 5

Turn the components into root stems where necessary.

1. gastro _______________________
2. dent _______________________
3. cephal _______________________
4. encephalo _______________________
5. gloss _______________________

6. tonsill _______________________
7. laryngo _______________________
8. cranio _______________________
9. chondr _______________________
10. bronchio _______________________

Solutions For Student Practice Activities

Activity 1

1. S	6. P	11. A	16. A
2. S	7. A	12. P	17. S
3. CF	8. P	13. S	18. CF
4. A	9. P	14. CF	19. A
5. S	10. S	15. P	20. A

Activity 2

1. D   2. F   3. C   4. A   5. E   6. B

Activity 3

1. gastro	6. chole
2. viri	7. tracheo
3. carpo	8. chondro
4. osteo	9. angio
5. genu	10. entero

Activity 4

1. glosso
3. esophago
4. stomato
7. chondro
8. myoso

Activity 5

1. gastr
4. encephal
7. laryng
8. crani
10. bronchi

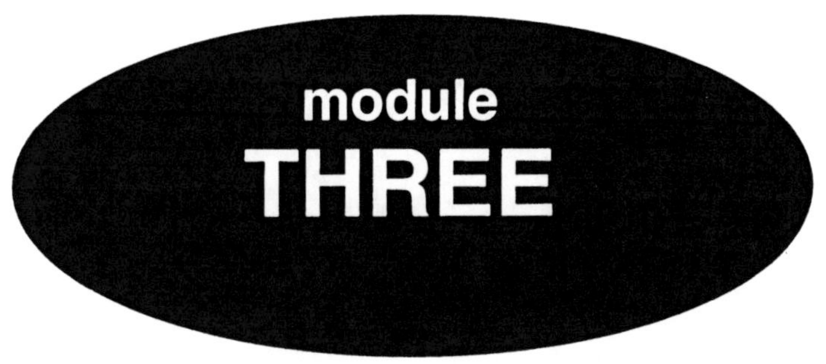

Rules of Combining

Objectives

Upon completion of this module the student should be able to:

1. Construct a correctly spelled medical term by selecting the proper components for the medical sentence.

2. Use the appropriate rules of combining to form a correctly spelled medical term.

3. Use the rules for analyzing a medical term to determine the definition of the word(s).

4. Correctly complete the activity portion of this module.

Component Combining Rules

A. Combining form(s)/Root Stem(s) attaches to a suffix

1. If suffix begins with a vowel, drop the combining vowel from the combining form and attach the suffix.

myo (muscles)	+	–itis	my	+ –itis	myitis
gastro (stomach)	+	–algia (pain)	gastr	+ –algia	gastralgia

2. If suffix begins with a consonant, leave the combining vowel in place and combine as is.

nephro (kidney)	+	–pexy (surgical suspension)	nephropexy
stomato (mouth)	+	–megaly	stomatomegaly

3. If suffix begins with a vowel and attaches to a root stem, combine as is.

cephal (head)	+	–oma (tumor)	cephaloma
arthr (joint)	+	–itis	arthritis

4. If suffix begins with a consonant and attaches to root stem, the combining vowel must be added. All anatomic roots/root stems have an assigned combining vowel whether it appears on the component or not; the vowel is usually "o".

rhin (nose)	+ –plasty (surgical reconstruction)		rhino	+ –plasty	rhinoplasty
cephal (head)	+ –megaly		cephalo	+ –megaly	cephalomegaly

5. If the combining form ends in two (2) vowels, and the suffix begins with a vowel, follow A.1.—drop the combining vowel from the combining form and attach the suffix.

   Remember only the last vowel is the combining vowel; the vowel preceding the combining vowel is part of the root stem.

cardio (heart)	+	–ac (pertaining to)	cardi	+	–ac	cardiac
osteo (bone)	+	–otomy (incision into)	oste	+	–otomy	osteotomy

6. If the vowel at the end of the root stem is to combine with a suffix starting with the same vowel the two like vowels may be combined. Both spellings are equally correct. Using both like vowels is considered the formal spelling; the contracted form is the more usual informal spelling.

   In some words common usage has caused these vowels to always combine. This only pertains to the joining of a combining form/root stem with a suffix.

cardio (heart)	+	–itis	cardiitis or carditis (formal) (informal)
osteo (bone)	+	–ectomy	osteectomy or ostectomy

7. If the combining form ends in two (2) vowels and the suffix begins with a consonant, combine following A.2.

osteo	+	–malacia (softening of)	osteomalacia
cranio (skull)	+	–cele (herniation)	craniocele

B. Prefix Combining

Prefixes are components which are attached to the beginning of a word, to a root form or suffix, without change in spelling of either component. The vowel found at the end of some prefixes is not a combining vowel.

1.

Prefix	+	*Suffix*	*Term Formed*
poly–	+	–phagia	polyphagia
di–	+	–uresis (urination)	diuresis
eu–	+	–pnea (breathing)	eupnea
dys–	+	–orexia (appetite)	dysorexia

2. *Prefix*	+	*Combining Form*	+	*Suffix*	*Term Formed*
peri–	+	gastro	+	–ic	perigastric
hemi–	+	esophago (esophagus)	+	–algia	hemiesophagalgia
pan–	+	myo	+	–dynia	panmyodynia
tachy–	+	cardio	+	–ia	tachycardia
post–	+	urethro (urethra)	+	–al	posturethral

C. Combining Multiple Root Forms

When combining more than one root word/combining forms together, all remain intact each with its combining vowel in place until the combining form that attaches to the suffix, then rules of section A.1. above are followed. Placement of combining forms in a word usually follows the flow of or adjoining structures.

1. *Multiple Combining Forms*   + *Suffix*   *Term Formed*

stomato + dento + glosso + –plasty
        (teeth) (tongue)

                        stomatodentoglossoplasty

broncho + tracheo + –plegia
(bronchus) (trachea)

                      bronchotracheoplegia
                      tracheobronchoplegia

2. A hyphen may be used between combining forms when the attached combining forms start with a vowel. There is no firm rule governing this; the appearance of the word to the eye and the attempt to highlight and clarify the spelling of each component within the word allows the choice. This rule does NOT apply when joining a combining form to a suffix.

Combining Forms   + *Suffix*   *Term Formed*

gastro + entero + colo + –itis   gastroenterocolitis
                                gastro-enterocolitis

tracheo + esophago + –odynia
                            tracheoesophagodynia
                            tracheo-esophagodynia

3. A root stem must be changed to a combining form before joining to another combining form.

Root Stems/Anatomic Roots   + *Suffix*   *Term Formed*

my	+	tendin	+	arthr	+	–ectomy
myo	+	tendino	+	arthro	+	–ectomy
		(tendon)				

                        myotendinoarthrectomy
                        myotendino-arthrectomy

Root Stems/Anatomic Roots				+ *Suffix*	*Term Formed*
cardi	+	angi	+	–pathy	
cardio	+	angio	+	–pathy	
		(vessel)			

cardioangiopathy cardio-angiopathy

Analyzing Medical Terms

To determine the meaning of the components within a word, the definition of that word is formed.

1. Read the word/term.

2. Divide it into its components.

3. Define each component.

4. Start with the definition of the suffix, go to prefix and then to the combining form(s).

5. By putting these definitions together in sentence form the meaning of the word/term.

EXAMPLE 1:

1.	TERM:	glossopharyngitis
2.		glosso/pharyng/itis
3.		tongue/throat/inflammation
4.		inflammation / the tongue / throat
5.		inflammation of the tongue and throat

EXAMPLE 2:

1.	TERM:	cephalalgia
2.		cephal/algia
3.		head/pain
4.		pain in / head
5.		pain in the head; headache

EXAMPLE 3:

1.	TERM:	perigastroenteritis
2.		peri/gastro/enter/itis
3.		around/stomach/intestines/inflammation
4.		inflammation / around / the stomach / intestines
5.		inflammation around the stomach and intestines

Word Synthesis

To build a word from a sentence:

1. Read the sentence carefully.

2. Select the components necessary to build the word.

3. Place the components in the proper order for combining.

4. Use the "Rules of Combining" to join components to form a correctly spelled word.

EXAMPLE 1:

1. Sentence: pain in all the muscle(s) and joint(s)

2. Selecting components:

<pre>
pain in / all / muscle(s) / joint(s)
–algia   pan–   myo   arthro
–dynia   pan–   myo   arthro
</pre>

3. Place in proper order:

prefix		*combining forms*			*suffix*
pan–	+	myo	+	arthro	+	–algia
pan–	+	myo	+	arthro	+	–dynia

4. Combine: see rules for combining prefix + multiple combining forms + suffix beginning with a vowel or consonant

prefix		*combining form*		*root stem*		*suffix*
pan–	+	myo	+	arthr	+	–algia
pan–	+	myo	+	arthr	+	–dynia

Word Constructed:

panmyoarthralgia   or panmyo-arthralgia   or panarthromyalgia
panmyoarthrodynia or panmyo-arthrodynia or panarthromyodynia

EXAMPLE 2:

1. "inflammation of the kidney"

2. inflammation of / the kidney
           –itis   nephro

3. nephro + –itis

4. nephr + –itis

    Word Constructed: nephritis

EXAMPLE 3:

1. "difficulty breathing"

2. difficulty/breathing

3. dys + –pnea

    Word Constructed: dyspnea

Student Practice Activities

Combining Components to Form Words

Activity 1

Attaching a combining form to a suffix which starts with a vowel (see A.1.)

1. myo   +   –oma   _______________________________
2. stomato +   –ectasis _______________________________
3. arthro   +   –itis   _______________________________
4. gastro   +   –algia   _______________________________
5. osteo   +   –otomy   _______________________________

Activity 2

Attaching a combining form to a suffix which starts with consonant (see A.2.)

1. chondro +   –malacia _______________________________
2. cephalo +   –megaly   _______________________________
3. cardio   +   –plasty   _______________________________
4. entero   +   –plegia   _______________________________
5. nephro   +   –ptosis   _______________________________

Activity 3

Attaching a root stem/anatomic root to a suffix which begins with a vowel (see A.3.)

1. enter   +   –ectasis _______________________________
2. col   +   –ostomy   _______________________________

Activity 3

(continued)

3. cephal + –otomy _______________________

4. esophag + –oma _______________________

5. stomat + –itis _______________________

Activity 4

Attaching a root stem/anatomic root to a suffix which begins with a consonant (see A.4.)

1. gastr + –genic _______________________

2. nephr + –gram _______________________

3. dent + –lysis _______________________

4. esophag + –sarcoma _______________________

5. my + –plasm _______________________

Activity 5

Attaching a combining form which ends in two vowels to a suffix which starts with a vowel (see A.5.)

1. osteo + –algia _______________________

2. cardio + –otomy _______________________

3. tracheo + –ostomy _______________________

4. cranio + –ectomy _______________________

5. angio + –oma _______________________

Activity 6

Attaching a combining form which ends in two vowels to a suffix which starts with a consonant (see A.7.)

1. osteo + –malacia _______________
2. cardio + –megaly _______________
3. tracheo + –spasm _______________
4. cranio + –plasty _______________
5. angio + –lysis _______________

Activity 7

Attaching a root stem/anatomic root ending with a vowel to any suffix (see A.5., A.6., A.7.)

1. angi + –ectasis _______________
2. cardi + –megalia _______________
3. oste + –otomy _______________
4. trache + –stenosis _______________
5. arteri + –sclerosis _______________

Activity 8

Attaching prefixes (see B.1.)

1. auto– + –phagia _______________
2. dys– + –uria _______________
3. poly– + –spasm _______________
4. hemi– + –plegia _______________
5. brady– + –cardia _______________

Activity 9

Combining multiple root forms (see C.1., 2. and 3.)

1. myo + tendino + chondro + –malacia

_____________________________ or _____________________________

or _____________________________

2. entero + colo + –itis

_____________________________ or _____________________________

3. tracheo + broncho + –stenosis

_____________________________ or _____________________________

4. cardio + angio + –spasm

_____________________________ or _____________________________

5. stomato + dento + –plasty

_____________________________ or _____________________________

Activity 10

Combining prefix, combining form(s) and suffix

1. peri– + dento + gingivo + –itis

_____________________________ or _____________________________

2. oligo– + leuko + –cytes

____

Activity 10 (continued)

3. supra– + reno + –al
     (kidney)

____

4. hemi– + encephalo + –ectomy
     (brain)

____

5. poly– + osteo + arthro + –oma

______________________ or ______________________

Activity 11

Analyzing Medical Terms (See page 22)

1. chondrectomy ______________________

____

2. osteochondromalacia ______________________

____

3. stomatodentoplasty ______________________

____

4. perimyoarthralgia ______________________

____

Activity 11

Analyzing Medical Terms (continued)

5. cephaloencephalomegalia _______________________________

____

6. eupnea ____

____

Activity 12

Word synthesis – building medical terms   (See pages 22–23)

1. Surgical removal of the stomach

____

2. Temporary opening into the cranium

____

3. Dilatation of all the stomach and intestines

____

4. Pain in the throat and esophagus
    (pharyngo)

____

5. Incision around a tendon and joint

____

Activity 12

Word synthesis – building medical terms (continued)

6. No feeling

____

7. One side

____

8. Difficulty swallowing

____

Solutions for Student Practice Activities

Activity 1

1. myoma
2. stomatectasis
3. arthritis
4. gastralgia
5. osteotomy

Activity 2

1. chondromalacia
2. cephalomegaly
3. cardioplasty
4. enteroplegia
5. nephroptosis

Activity 3

1. enterectasis
2. colostomy
3. cephalotomy
4. esophagoma
5. stomatitis

Activity 4

1. gastrogenic
2. nephrogram
3. dentolysis
4. esophagosarcoma
5. myoplasm

Activity 5

1. ostealgia
2. cardiotomy
3. tracheostomy
4. craniectomy
5. angioma

Activity 6

1. osteomalacia
2. cardiomegaly
3. tracheospasm
4. cranioplasty
5. angiolysis

Activity 7

1. angiectasis
2. cardiomegalia
3. osteotomy
4. tracheostenosis
5. arteriosclerosis

Activity 8

1.autophagia
2.dysuria
3.polyspasm
4.hemiplegia
5.bradycardia

Activity 9

1. myotendinochondromalacia
   tendinochondromyomalacia
   chondromyotendinomalacia

2. enterocolitis
   coloenteritis

3. tracheobronchostenosis
   bronchotracheostenosis

4. cardioangiospasm
   angiocardiospasm
   cardio-angiospasm

5. stomatodentoplasty
   dentostomatoplasty

Activity 10

1. peridentogingivitis
   perigingivodentitis

2. oligoleukocytes

3. suprarenal

4. hemiencephalectomy

5. polyosteoarthroma
   polyosteo-arthroma
   polyarthroosteoma
   polyarthro-osteoma

Activity 11

1. excision of cartilage
   surgical removal of cartilage

2. softening of cartilage and bone(s)

3. surgical reconstruction of the mouth and teeth
   plastic repair of the mouth and teeth

4. pain around the muscle(s) and joint(s)

5. enlarged head and brain
   large head and brain

6. normal breathing

Activity 12

1. gastrectomy

2. craniotomy

3. pangastroenterectasis
   pangastro-enterectasis

4. pharyngo-esophagalgia
   pharyngoesophagalgia
   pharyngo-esophagodynia
   pharyngoesophagodynia

5. peritendino-arthrotomy
   periarthrotendinotomy

6. anesthesia

7. hemilateral, unilateral

8. dysphagia

Irregularities in Word/Component Formation
Exceptions to the Rules

A. Irregularities

Irregularities in the formation of prefix/combining form/suffix components.

1. Some components, regardless of their type, will automatically join together when they are in the same word regardless of their type. Usually they form a new suffix. These components never separate into their usual placement. These newly formed components may, also, be used as words; the definition remains the same.

EXAMPLES:

Component		*Suffix*	*New Suffix/Word*
litho (stone[s])	+	–otomy	–lithotomy (incision for the removal of stone[s]) lithotomy (word)
litho	+	–iasis	–lithiasis lithiasis (word)
endo–	+	–scope	–endoscope endoscope (word)
endo–	+	–scopy	–endoscopy endoscopy (word)

2. With increasing frequency of usage, new suffixes are being formed and are used as words and suffixes, but these are not consistent in their formation.

EXAMPLE:

Component		*Suffix*	*New Suffix/Word*
a–, an–	+	–trophy	–atrophy atrophy (word)
hyper–	+	–esthesia	–hyperesthesia hyperesthesia (word)
a–, an–	+	–sthenia	–asthenia asthenia (word)

3. Some components and combinations of components have become permanently established terms in our vocabulary. When defining, the individual component definitions are not considered separately but are considered as a new word with its own specific meaning. Most have been accepted as words as well as suffixes.

EXAMPLES:

anastomosis	hyperesthesia
asthenia	lithiasis
carcinoma	lithotomy
edema	sarcoma

        emesis   sclerosis
        endoscope   stenosis
        endoscopy

B. Noun Suffix

A **noun suffix** is formed when the root stem is joined to a noun ending. This newly formed suffix is used at the end of a word instead of the usual suffix. It gives the root stem the meaning of "condition of having a condition or disease".

EXAMPLE:

Root Stem	*+*	*Noun Ending*	*Noun Suffix*
cardi	+	–ia	–cardia
encephal	+	–on	–encephalon
arthr	+	–ia	–arthria

C. Root Words

Root words having more than one combining form.

There is no set rule controlling this group of components. Each is considered individually.

1. stomato/stoma

   stomato is the preferred combining form for the oral mouth, e.g., stomatitis

   stoma is used to indicate "a mouthlike opening created surgically." It is used as a word or suffix, e.g., the stoma of the colostomy. Rarely is stoma used to indicate the oral mouth.

2. myo/myoso

   Both forms have the same meaning and are interchangeable when forming words, e.g., myalgia or myosalgia.

3. glyco/glycoso

   Both components will combine with any and all suffixes except –uria. –uria will only combine with "glycoso", e.g.,

glyco/glycoso	+	–emia	glycemia or glycosemia
glyco/glycoso	+	–uria	glycosuria only

4. hemo/hemato; dermo/dermato; chromo/chromato

   hemo, dermo and chromo always combine with suffixes starting with a consonant.

   hemato, dermato and chromato always combine with suffixes starting with a vowel.

   The dictionary and common usage will show words that do not follow this rule, but when uncertain the application of this rule is standard. Example: hemopoiesis or hematopoiesis — both are found in the dictionary.

This rule does not apply when combining with another combining form or with a noun suffix.

Example: hemo, hemato + chromato + –osis

           hemochromatosis
           hematochromatosis

When affixed before another combining form either form may be used.

Example: hemo, hemato   + –ptysis   hemoptysis
hemo, hemato   + –oma   hematoma

The exceptional exception:

hemo/hemato   + –crit   hematocrit — only

D. Suffix

Suffix – exceptions to the rule of joining a combining form with a suffix.

1. Some suffixes consistently combine without dropping the combination bowel. Each is also used as a word.

  -endoscopy
  thoraco + -endoscopy thoracoendoscopy

  -endoscope
  cardio + -endoscope cardioendoscope

  -anastomosis
  gastro + -anastomosis gastroanastomosis

  -ankylosis
  arthro + -ankylosis   arthroankylosis

2. **"-atresia"** and **"-edema"** combine with combining forms either by retaining or dropping the combining vowel of the combining form, whichever is your preference.

EXAMPLES:

  myo   + -edema   myoedema or myedema

  esophago + -atresia   esophagoatresia or esophagatresia

E. Prefixes — exceptions:

1. **oligo–** Although this component is a prefix, it follows the rules for combining forms. It is NOT a combining form, therefore, it will always appear at the beginning of a word.

EXAMPLE:

Prefix	+	*Combining Form*	+	*Suffix*	*Term*
oligo–	+	–dipsia			oligodipsia
oligo–	+	erythro	+	–cytes	oligoerythrocytes
oligo–	+	–uria			oliguria
oligo–			+	-cmia	oligemia

2. **para–** Words starting with "para–" frequently can not be defined using the established rules. A dictionary should be consulted to determine the meaning of the word and how para combines with other components.

   Because this component has such a variety of meanings, it is difficult to define the word in which it is a part, e.g., paralysis: adjacent or near breakdown or freeing-up; beyond breakdown or freeing-up. None of these definitions make sense.

   "para–" also is not consistent in following the rules of combining. With some components it always follows the rule for prefixes, as with paralysis; or it may follow the exception to the rule as does "oligo-" and drops the final vowel as in "parenteral" or "paresthesia". With some other components it combines using either of these rules, with or without the final vowel as in paraurethral or parurethral.

3. **"micro–"** and **"macro"** are undergoing the same change of combining structure. The alternative spelling is seen in scientific tracts as well as in rarely used forms of medical terminology: micrelectrical, macrophthalmos, micrencephaly.

   Because of these variations in spelling when using these prefixes ending in a vowel joining combining form or a noun suffix starting with a vowel, it is best to check the dictionary when unsure.

4. **a-, an-**   These prefixes follow the rule for usage as in everyday speech.

   "a-" is attached to components starting with a consonant:

a-	+		-pnea	apnea
a-	+		-phagia	aphagia

   "an-" is attached to components starting with a vowel:

an-	+		-uria	anuria
an-	+		-esthesia	anesthesia

In speaking we say: an apple or a book. It is rare that one hears the misuse of this prefix, even from children.

The formation of a new component may occur when either two combining forms or a prefix and combining form join to create a new combining form. As with any term the newly formed component now conveys a specific idea that is distinctly different from its individual parts.

EXAMPLE:

Combining Forms			*New Component Forms*
chole (bile)	+	angio (vessel, duct)	cholangio (bile duct)
peri- (around)	+	osteo (bone)	periosteo (the membrane covering the bone)
myo (muscle)	+	metrio (uterus)	myometrio (muscle of the uterus)

F. Use of –ostomy and –anastomosis

–ostomy is defined as a more or less permanent opening when combined with one combining form indicating one anatomical structure has an opening. If more than one combining form (tubular anatomical structures) are affixed before –ostomy, it has the same meaning as anastomosis, or forming a communication between these structures.

EXAMPLE:

Components	*Term*
colo + –ostomy (large intestines)	colostomy (a more or less permanent opening made in the intestines)
entero + colo + –ostomy (intestines)	enterocolostomy (creating a communication between the large and small intestines)
entero + colo + –anastomosis	enterocoloanastomosis (creating a communication between the large and small intestines)

NOTE: "entero" is defined as intestines — any part of the intestinal tract; only when combining with "colo" is it defined as the small intestine.

G. Rule of "X" — Forming combining forms from words ending in "x".

Words ending in "x" cannot be used as combining forms; they must be changed to a root stem, then to a combining form before another component, combining form or suffix, is attached.

1. If the letter preceding the "x" is a vowel, the "x" is dropped and is replaced by "c". This forms the root stem; a combining vowel — usually "o" is attached to form the combining form.

EXAMPLE:

Word	*Root Stem*	*Combining Form*
thorax	thorac	thoraco
cervix	cervic	cervico

2. If the letter preceding the "x" is an "e", there as an additional change. The "e" becomes an "i" and the "x" becomes "c".

EXAMPLE:

Word	*Root Stem*	*Combining Form*
apex	apic	apico
index	indic	indico

3. If the letter preceding the "x" is a consonant the "x" is dropped and is replaced by "g". This forms the root stem. A combining vowel is attached to form the combining form.

EXAMPLE:

Word	*Root Stem*	*Combining Form*
larynx	laryng	laryngo
pharynx	pharyng	pharyngo

4. If the letter preceding the "x" is a "y", the "y" is usually considered a consonant, but not always. Fortunately there are not many words ending in "–yx". The two examples included appear most frequently as medical terms. Because the "y" in calyx functions as an "i", this word is spelled with either "y" or "i" and is correct with either spelling.

EXAMPLE:

Word	*Root Stem*	*Combining Form*
calyx, calix	calyc, calic	calyco, calico
coccyx	coccyg	coccygo

The plural forms of words apex and index may appear as apexes and indexes. This may be considered acceptable but not proper word formation, much like "ain't" is accepted but considered as nonstand ard word usage.

5. Words ending in "x" being used as a noun suffix usually maintain the "x". The plural forms maintain their usual plural ending. As with any language there are exceptions to the rules which are just as absolute as the basic rules.

Student Practice Activities for Exceptions and Irregularities

Apply the rules of combining for the following problems. Do not attempt to define the words formed.

1. oligo-   +   -emia

2. oligo-   +   -pnea

3. oligo-   +   -genic

4. oligo-   +   -uria

5. a-, an-   +   encephalo   +   -ous

6. a-, an-   +   -genic

7. a-, an-   +   myo   +   -plasia

8. a-, an-   +   -uresis

9. a-, an-   +   -phasia

10. a-, an-   +   -emia

11. nephro   +   litho   +   -iasis

12. cranio + -scopy ____

13. entero + gastro + -anastomosis _______________________________

14. myo, myoso + -edema ____

15. esophago + -atresia ____

16. thoraco + endo- + -scope ____

17. nephro + litho + -otomy ____

18. rhino + litho + -iasis ____

19. glyco, glycoso + -penia ____

20. a-, an- + -esthesia ____

21. glyco, glycoso + -uria ____

22. hemo, hemato + -ptysis ____

23. dermo, dermato + -itis ____

24. hemo, hemato + -oma ____

25. dermo, dermato +   -lysis _______________________________

26. peri-   +   cranio   +   -ia _______________________________

*27. intra-   +   thorax _______________________________

28. salpinx   +   -itis _______________________________

29. hemo, hemato   +   -emesis _______________________________

*30. thorax   +   -otomy _______________________________

31. hemi-   +   encephalo   +   -on _______________________________

*32. coccyx   +   -es _______________________________

*33. apex   +   -al _______________________________

*34. pharynx   +   -anastomosis _______________________________

35. a-, an-   +   -sthenia _______________________________

*36. hemo, hemato   +   thoraco _______________________________

*Remember to review Rule of X

Solutions for Practice Activities for Exceptions and Irregularities

1. oligemia
2. oligopnea
3. oligogenic
4. oliguria
5. anencephalous
6. agenic
7. amyoplasia
8. anuresis
9. aphasia
10. anemia
11. nephrolithiasis
12. cranioscopy
13. enterogastroanastomosis
    gastro-enteroanastomosis
    gastroenteroanastomosis
14. myoedema, myedema
    myosoedema, myosedema
15. esophagatresia
    esophagoatresia
16. thoracoendoscope
17. nephrolithotomy
18. rhinolithiasis
19. glycosopenia, glycopenia
20. anesthesia
21. glycosuria
22. hemoptysis
23. dermatitis
24. hematoma
25. dermolysis
26. pericrania
27. intrathorax
28. salpingitis
29. hematemesis
30. thoracotomy
31. hemiencephalon
32. coccyges
33. apical
34. pharyngoanastomosis
35. asthenia
36. hemothorax

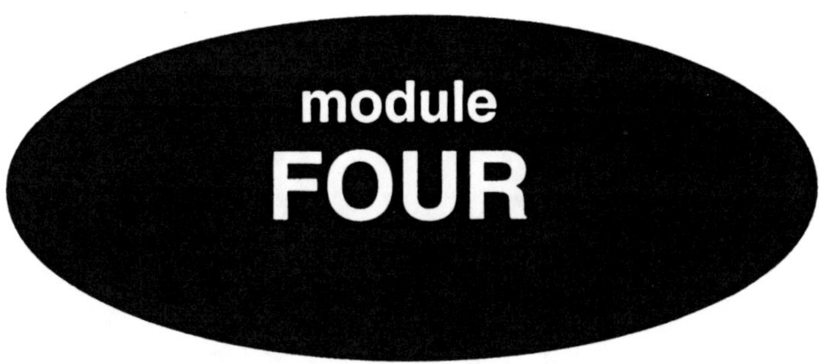

Suffixes

Objectives

Upon completion of this module the student should be able to:

1. Identify and differentiate prefixes, suffixes, root stems and combining forms.

2. Write the correctly spelled component, given a list of definitions.

3. Write the definitions for each, given a list of components.

4. Divide the medical term(s) into individual appropriate components; using these definitions, construct a sentence to define the word.

5. Assign the appropriate components to build a medical term when given a medical sentence and construct a correctly spelled medical term.

6. Complete all activities in this module correctly.

A. Suffixes

Definition: A *suffix* is a component which tells what is happening in a word. A hyphen is placed in front of the component to indicate a suffix always comes at the end of the word. Spelling never changes when combined with other components. A few suffixes have come into the language as words. Some have more than one spelling.

Suffix	*Meaning of Suffix*
1. –algia	a. pain
2. –carcinoma (carcinoma)*	a. *malignant tumor* of *epithelial* tissue b. *cancer* of epithelial tissue: tissue that lines or covers the body organs or body cavities; the skin
3. –cele	a. *herniation:* abnormal protrusion of an organ or tissue through a defect or any normal opening of the body
4. –centesis	a. puncture for *aspiration* b. puncture for removal of any body fluid or air by suction c. tapping for drainage
5. –clasis	a. surgical fracture
6. –desis	a. surgical binding (pertains to connective tissue)
7. –dipsia	a. thirst
8. –dynia	a. pain
9. –ectasis –ectasia	a. dilation b. stretching open c. distention

Note: ( )* indicate usage of component as a word.
 Italicized words are defined in Vocabulary.

Suffix		*Meaning of Suffix*
10. –ectomy	a.	surgical removal
	b.	*excision* of
	c.	cutting out
11. –emia	a.	present in the bloodstream
12. –emesis	a.	vomiting
(emesis)	b.	to vomit
13. –endoscope	a.	instrument used to inspect body cavities
14. –endoscopy	a.	procedure using an instrument to inspect body cavities
15. –esthesia	a.	feeling
(esthesia)	b.	sensation
	c.	perception
16. –genic	a.	originating
	b.	origin
	c.	producing
17. –gram	a.	a recorded, written record or picture (X–ray)
	b.	a recorded picture or record (is visible or written)
electro– (root word) –gram	a.	a tracing of electrical activity of body activity
18. –graph	a.	instrument for making a written record, tracing or picture
	b.	instrument to record
19. –graphy	a.	process of recording
	b.	making a tracing or picture
20. –iasis	a.	presence of (implies presence of foreign matter)
	b.	condition of having
21. –itis	a.	*inflammation* of
	b.	inflammatory process: tissues are red, hot, swollen with pain and/or itching
22. –lithiasis	a.	presence of stone(s) in body; presence of calculus (calculi)
(lithiasis)		
23. –lithotomy	a.	incision for removal of stone(s)
(lithotomy)		
24. –lysis	a.	dissolution, decomposition
(lysis)	b.	breakdown
	c.	freeing up
	d.	relief of
25. –malacia	a.	softening of
(malacia)		

Suffix	*Meaning of Suffix*
26. –megaly –megalia	a. enlargement of b. large c. enlarged
27. –oid	a. resembling b. like
28. –oma	a. *tumor* (–oma may denote a benign or cancerous tumor)
29. –ology	a. study of
30. –ostomy	a. more or less permanent opening (ostomy) b. artificial surgical opening c. *anastomosis:* joining two or more cavities or tubular structures to allow a continuous flow d. joining of two or more tubular structures to allow a continuous flow
31. –osis	a. abnormal condition b. increase in condition
32. –otomy	a. *incision* into, of, or for b. temporary opening c. cutting into, of or for
33. –paresis (paresis)	a. weakness
34. –pathy	a. disease
35. –penia	a. deficiency b. decrease c. poverty
36. –pepsia	a. digestion
37. –pexy	a. surgical suspension (pertains to nonepithelial connective tissue or internal organs)
38. –phagia	a. swallowing b. swallow c. eating
39. –phasia	a. speech–coherence and verbal comprehension b. ability to communicate using words
40. –phonia	a. voice b. vocal sounds c. sounds of speech
41. –plasia –plasm	a. tissue formation (affects number of cells)
42. –plakia	a. patches, plaques
43. –plasty	a. plastic repair b. surgical reconstruction

Suffix		*Meaning of Suffix*

44. –plegia   a. paralysis: inability to move voluntarily

45. –pnea
   a. breathe
   b. breathing
   c. breath

46. –ptosis
    –ptosia
    (ptosis)
   a. downward displacement
   b. prolapse
   c. drooping
   d. floating

47. –ptysis
    (ptysis)
   a. spitting
   b. expectorating

48. –rrhage
    –rrhagia
   a. bleeding
   b. abnormal flow (usually refers to blood)
   c. abnormal discharge of blood (rapid discharge)

49. –rrhea
   a. flow of any fluid except blood or pus
   b. discharge (usually not blood)

50. –rrhaphy
   a. suture
   b. surgical repair
   c. to sew

51. –rrhexis   a. rupture: abrupt separation of tissue

52. –sarcoma
    (sarcoma)
   a. malignant tumor of connective tissue
   b. cancer of non–epithelial tissue
   c. malignancy of fleshy tissue

53. –sclerosis
    (sclerosis)
   a. hardening of

54. –scope
    (scope)
   a. instrument used for viewing or examining
   b. instrument to look through when viewing or examining

55. –scopy
   a. procedure using an instrument for viewing or examining

56. –spasm
    (spasm)
   a. involuntary contractions
   b. uncontrolled contractions

57. –stenosis
    (stenosis)
   a. narrowing of

58. –sthenia   a. strength

59. –tasis   a. stretching

60. –therapy
    (therapy)
   a. treatment

61. –trophy   a. cell nourishment (affects size of cells)

62. –uria
   a. present in the urine
   b. pertaining to urine

Suffix		*Meaning of Suffix*
63. –uresis (uresis)	a. b. c.	urination passage of urine voiding

Adjective Suffixes		*Meaning of Suffix*
Example		
64. -ac, -al, -ar, -ary, -ic	a. b. c.	pertaining to having to do with concerning
65. –ism	a. b.	characteristic of having to do with
66. –ous	a. b.	full of abundance of

Student Practice Activities – Suffixes

Activity 1

Flash Cards

Make a separate card for each suffix. Print the correctly spelled suffix on one side of the card and the definition on the opposite side. Make flash cards for italicized Vocabulary terms in the module; print the definition on the opposite side. Make sure each is correctly spelled.

Activity 2

Memorize all suffixes and words in this module.

Practice identifying/reciting/writing component definitions.

Practice identifying/reciting/writing correct component spelling each correctly.

Activity 3

Word Building and Defining (continued)

Follow instructions carefully to correctly complete these practice activities.

Note how by changing the suffix the meaning of the word changes. The following problems demonstrate how the definition of a word changes when the suffix is changed.

Combining Form	+ Suffix	Medical Term and Definition
Example:		
a. chondro (cartilage)	–plasty (surgical reconstruction)	chondroplasty (surgical reconstruction of cartilage)
b. chondro	–sarcoma (malignant tumor of non–epithelial tissue)	chondrosarcoma (malignant cartilage tumor)
c. myo (muscle)	–oma (tumor)	myoma (muscle tumor)
d. myo	–itis (inflammation of)	myitis (inflammation of muscle)
e. myelo (bone marrow)	–genic (producing of, originating in)	myelogenic (originating in bone marrow)
f. myelo	–centesis (puncture for aspiration)	myelocentesis (puncture for aspiration of bone marrow)

Using rules of Module 2 combine the following combining forms with suffixes to form correctly spelled medical terms. Write the medical term and a short definition.

Combining Form	Suffix	Medical Term	Definition
Example:			
arthro (joint)	–malacia	arthromalacia	softening of joint
1. arthro	–osis	_____________	_____________
2. arthro	–algia	_____________	_____________

Activity 3

Word Building and Defining (continued)

Combining Form	Suffix	Medical Term	Definition
3. arthro	–dynia		
4. arthro	–desis		
5. arthro	–otomy		
6. cranio (skull)	–otomy		
7. cranio	–plasty		
8. cranio	–malacia		
9. cranio	–cele		
10. cranio	–ectomy		
11. cranio	–ostomy		
12. chondro (cartilage)	–sclerosis		
13. chondro	–oma		
14. chondro	–sarcoma		
15. chondro	–plasty		
16. chondro	–lysis		
17. chondro	–oid		
18. myo (muscle)	–ectomy		
19. myo	–dynia		
20. myo	–rrhaphy		
21. myo	–plasty		
22. myo	–sarcoma		

Activity 3

Word Building and Defining (continued)

Combining Form	Suffix	Medical Term	Definition
23. myelo (bone marrow)	–itis		
24. myelo	–oma		
25. myelo	–sarcoma		
26. myelo	–centesis		
27. myelo	–pathy		
28. spondylo (vertebra, sing.) (vertebrae, pl.)	–itis		
29. spondylo	–osis		
30. spondylo	–therapy		
31. spondylo	–malacia		
32. spondylo	–algia		
33. spondylo	–desis		
34. rachio	–algia		
35. thoraco	–megalia		
36. hemo	–rrhage		
37. colo	–pexy		
38. esophago	–gram		
39. osteo	–clasis		
40. myo	–esthesia		

Suffix Crossword Puzzle

Activity 4

Complete puzzle by using the suffix clues provided. All clues are components from the suffix list, except 1 Across and 1 Down. SUGGESTION: USE PENCIL!

ACROSS

1. Married ladies title
5. inflammation
10. prolapse
11. abnormal flow (bloody)
13. stretch, stretching
16. vomiting
17. softening
18. machine for making tracing
19. concerning
20. herniation
24. pain
25. tumor
28. voice, sounds of speech
29. narrow
31. thirst
32. spitting
33. type of puzzle components
36. pain (not 24 across)
37. x-ray picture
38. patches or plaques
39. strength
40. breathing
41. permanent opening
42. rupture
45. large, enlarged
47. non-bloody flow
48. using an instrument for visual examination
50. breakdown
52. tissue formation
53. puncture for aspiration
55. pertaining to, concerning
56. study of
57. urination
58. in the blood
60. treatment
61. noun suffix ending
62. increase in disease, abnormal condition

DOWN

1. author's name
2. surgical removal
3. surgical binding
4. weakness
6. cell nourishment
7. involuntary muscle contraction
8. digestion
9. making a picture/tracing
12. suture, surgical repair
14. eating, swallowing
15. instrument used for visual examination
19. state of, characteristic of
20. malignancy of epithelial tissue
21. feeling, sensation
22. disease
23. speech coherence
25. resembling, like
26. decrease; deficiency
27. incision for removal of stones
29. hardening
30. incision into, of
32. surgical reconstruction
34. stretching open
35. in the urine
38. surgical suspension
43. variation of #11 across
44. malignancy of connective non-epithelial tissue
46. origin, originating
49. paralysis
51. presence of, condition of
54. pertaining to
56. abundance of, full of
59. pertaining to

Suffix Crossword Puzzle

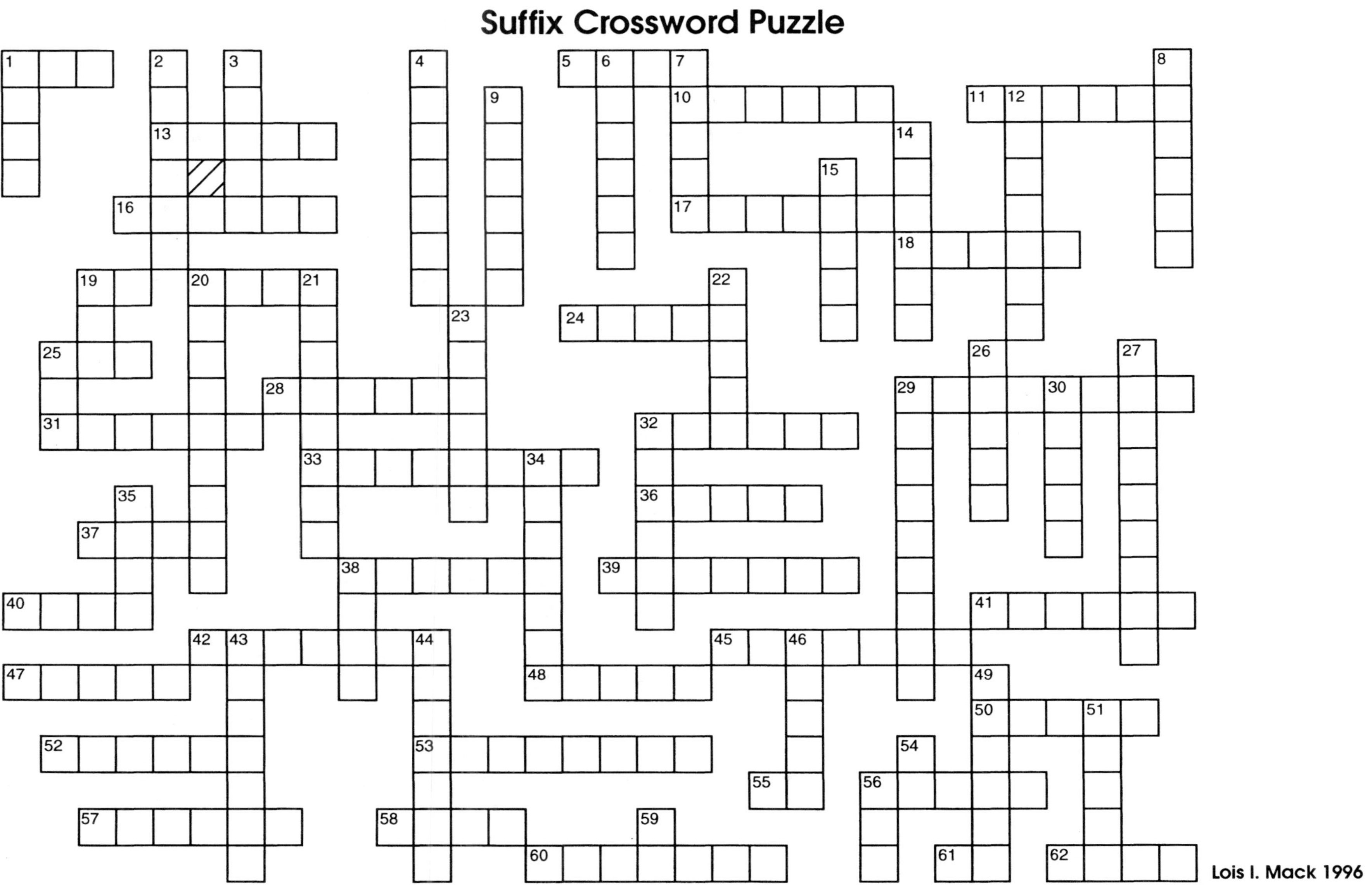

Lois I. Mack 1996

Medical Terminological Seek and Find

Activity 5

Look horizontally—left to right, vertically—top to bottom, or diagonally. Although there are 24 clues here are many other suffixes to be found.

Can You Find 24 Suffixes?

```
A I T I S L I S T H E S I S B C R R H A P H Y C O L M N O P N E A R S T
D I P S I A D R R H A P H Y L S T R G E C T O M Y P T A S I S E M E T A
D F E O T O M Y R M N P R R M W P T O S I S O S T O M Y S A R C O M E I
S G X A I N R H H O L L T O X E M I A A L M E R T E S I S P E X Y D E S
I H Y M O P E T E L A E V U T Y A T Y I T A C R U C W R U C C C C S U A
S I J O D A S R X K A G A B C Z L I L T A L A H K P L E G I A P A R E S
A M Y C Y O P R I J G I I L E K A S A I S A R E T R R H E X I S D I P S
M E M R N A B C S I E A S A H J C Y G S I C C X J Y X E P R R H S T I D
O G O A I D E F G H M G C D E F I M E Y S I I I Y P E N I A O D D E A L
N A T S A L G I A O S C O P Y Z A E M N C A N S U C A R C I N O M A L L
I L O S T O M Y H I K L P N O P L T I O T S T P S E M I L U N A R T K E
C Y A G B C D E F G S M E A B C O R R H A P H Y P O L Y D I U P S I A L M
R L G R A M A B D C I D E F S G T O I E M S R R Z O T H E R A P Y E A L
A A B A C D E F I A S I S I G H O R A M Y G G R R O S T O M Y P A N A R
C K H P A R G M O S C O P E R S M R S O O R R H Y U R I A U R E S I S T
A B C H G H I J K L M A W V U I Y H I T R A A E X D E S I S S C L E R O
D E F Y M O T O E C T A S I S S E E S S R M P A E S T E N O S I S P A N
O I D A B C D E S I S I J K L O N A Z O H W H H P A I G E L P P A R E S
I N T R A P L A S T Y E N D O P H A G I A P E R I I N T E R C E N T E S
C E L E P E R T U S S I S A N G I N A C E N T E S I S P H A S I A R S T
```

See if you can find more suffixes.

1. inflammation of
2. thirst
3. surgical suspension
4. surgical binding
5. suture
6. rupture
7. normal flow or discharge
8. paralysis
9. excision of
10. abnormal flow
11. incision; temporary opening
12. pain
13. anastomosis of
14. procedure for viewing
15. instrument for viewing
16. breathing
17. the process of recording
18. the instrument used for recording
19. the presence of
20. increase in; abnormal condition
21. stretching
22. enlargement of
23. malignant tumor
24. resembling

Solutions to Practice Activities

Activity 3

Word Building and Defining

1.	arthrosis	abnormal condition of joint(s)
2.	arthralgia	joint pain
3.	arthrodynia	joint pain
4.	arthrodesis	surgical binding of joint(s)
5.	arthrotomy	incision into joint(s)
6.	craniotomy	incision into the cranium (skull)
7.	cranioplasty	surgical reconstruction of the cranium, plastic repair of cranium
8.	craniomalacia	softening of the cranium
9.	craniocele	tissues herniating through a defect in the cranium
10.	craniectomy	surgical removal of part of the cranial bone (skull bone)
11.	craniostomy	to form a more or less permanent opening in the cranium
12.	chondrosclerosis	hardening of the cartilage
13.	chondroma	tumor of the cartilage
14.	chondrosarcoma	tumor of the cartilage
15.	chondroplasty	surgical reconstruction of the cartilage
16.	chondrolysis	breakdown of cartilage; freeing up cartilage
17.	chondroid	resembling cartilage
18.	myectomy	surgical excision of muscle
19.	myodynia	muscle pain
20.	myorrhaphy	suture of muscle(s), surgical repair of muscle(s)

Activity 3

Word Building and Defining (continued)

21.	myoplasty	plastic repair of muscle(s), surgical reconstruction of muscle(s)
22.	myosarcoma	malignant tumor of muscle, cancer of muscle
23.	myelitis	inflammation of bone marrow
24.	myeloma	tumor of bone marrow
25.	myelosarcoma	malignancy of bone marrow, cancer of bone marrow
26.	myelocentesis	puncture for aspiration of marrow
27.	myelopathy	disease of bone marrow
28.	spondylitis	inflammation of vertebra(e)
29.	spondylosis	abnormal condition of the vertebra(e)
30.	spondylotherapy	treatment to the vertebra(e)
31.	spondylomalacia	softening of the bones of vertebra(e)
32.	spondylalgia	pain in the vertebra(e)
33.	spondylodesis	binding of the vertebra(e)
34.	rachialgia	pain in the spinal column
35.	thoracomegaly	enlarged chest
36.	hemorrhagia	profuse flow of blood
37.	colopexy	suspension of the large intestine (colon)
38.	esophagogram	x-ray picture of the esophagus
39.	osteoclasis	surgical fracturing of bone(s)
40.	myesthesia	sensations of muscles contracting

Solutions to Activities – Suffixes

Activity 4

Suffixes Crossword Puzzle

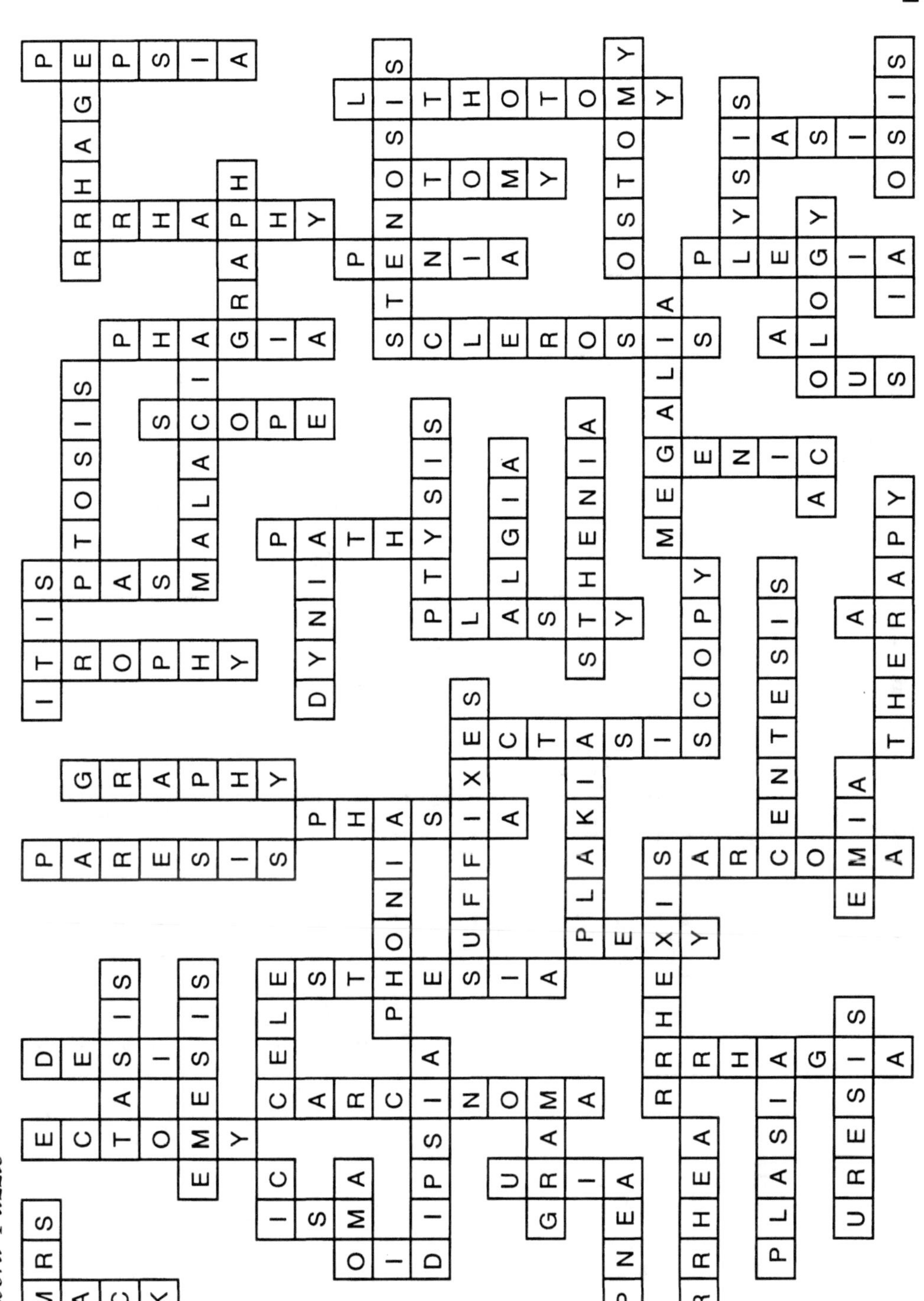

Solutions to Activities – Suffixes

Activity 5

Component Recognition: Seek and Find

Did You Find 24 Suffixes?

```
A I T I S L I S T H E S I S B C R R H A P H Y C O L M N O P N E A R S T
D I P S I A D R R H A P H Y L S T R G E C T O M Y P T A S I S E M E T A
D F E O T O M Y R M N P R R M W P T O S I S O S T O M Y S A R C O M E I
S G X A I N R H H O L L T O X E M I A A L M E R T E S I S P E X Y D E S
I H Y M O P E T E L A E V U T Y A T Y I T A C R U C W R U C C C S U A
S I J O D A S R X K A G A B C Z L I L T A L A H K P L E G I A P A R E S
A M Y C Y O P R I J G I I L E K A S A I S A R E T R R H E X I S D I P S
M E M R N A B C S I E A S A H J C Y G S I C C X J Y X E P R R H S T I D
O G O A I D E F G H M G C D E F I M E Y S I I I Y P E N I A O I D E A L
N A T S A L G I A O S C O P Y Z A E M N C A N S U C A R C I N O M A L L
I L O S T O M Y H I K L P N O P L T I O T S T P S E M I L U N A R T K E
C Y A G B C D E F G S M E A B C O R R H A P H Y P O L Y D I P S I A L M
R L G R A M A B D C I D E F S G T O I E M S R R Z O T H E R A P Y E A L
A A B A C D E F I A S I S I G H O R A M Y G G R R O S T O M Y P A N A R
C K H P A R G M O S C O P E R S M R S O O R R H Y U R I A U R E S I S T
A B C H G H I J K L M A W V U I Y H I T R A A E X D E S I S S C L E R O
D E F Y M O T O E C T A S I S E E S S R M P A E S T E N O S I S P A N
O I D A B C D E S I S I J K L O N A Z O H W H H P A I G E L P P A R E S
I N T R A P L A S T Y E N D O P H A G I A P E R I I N T E R C E N T E S
C E L E P E R T U S S I S A N G I N A C E N T E S I S P H A S I A R S T
```

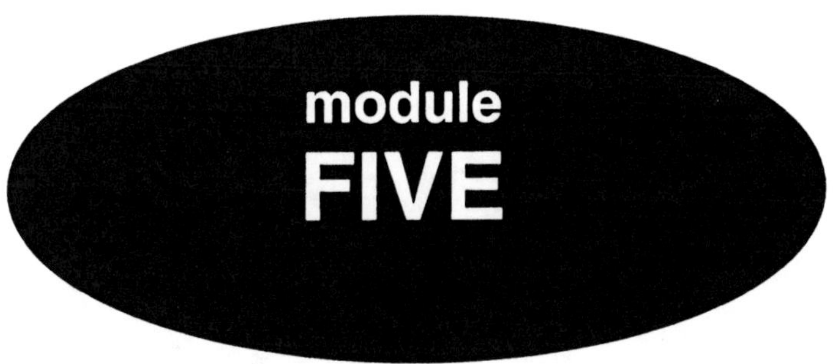

Prefixes

Objectives

Upon completion of this module the student should be able to:

1. Identify and differentiate prefixes, suffixes, root stems and combining forms.

2. Write the correctly spelled component, given a list of definitions.

3. Write the definitions for each, given a list of components.

4. Divide the medical term(s) into individual appropriate components; using these definitions, construct a sentence to define the word.

5. Assign the appropriate components to build a medical term when given a medical sentence and construct a correctly spelled medical term..

6. Complete all activities in this module correctly.

A. Prefixes

Definition: A *prefix* is a component placed at the beginning of a word affixed to a combining form or suffix. It does not change the meaning of the word but does modify the meaning as to amount, time, place, etc. Prefixes do not change spelling when combined.

Prefix	*Meaning of Prefix*
1. a-, (affix to component starting with a consonant) an-, (affix to component starting with a vowel)	a. not b. without c. absent d. absence of
2. ab-	a. away from
3. ad-	a. toward, to
4. ante-	a. before
5. anti-	a. against b. opposed
6. auto-	a. self
7. brady-	a. slow
8. con- com- (affix to components beginning with b, p, m)	a. with b. together c. in association with
9. contra-	a. against b. opposite
10. dextro-	a. to the right b. on the right side
11. dys-	a. bad b. difficult c. painful

Prefix	*Meaning of Prefix*
12. ecto-	a. outside (normal location) b. external
13. endo-	a. within b. inner
14. epi-	a. upon b. over (position)
15. eu-	a. healthy b. normal c. good d. well
16. ex-	a. out of b. from
17. extra-	a. outside of b. in addition to
18. hemi-	a. half (right or left side)
19. homo-	a. same
20. hyper-	a. excessive b. increase c. more than normal d. above
21. hypo-	a. less than b. decrease c. less than normal d. below e. under
22. infra-	a. below (located below another structure)
23. inter-	a. between
24. intra-	a. within b. inside
25. latero-	a. side
26. macro-	a. large
27. micro-	a. small
28. neo-	a. new
29. oligo-	a. scant b. few c. a little
30. pan-	a. all b. every c. total

Prefix	*Meaning of Prefix*
31. para-	a. near b. beside c. adjacent to d. beyond
32. peri-	a. around b. surrounding
33. poly-	a. many (more than normal) b. much (more than normal)
34. post-	a. behind b. after c. later
35. pro-	a. before b. in favor of c. forward
36. pseudo-	a. false
37. recti-	a. straight
38. retro-	a. behind b. backward
39. semi-	a. half (partial amount) (used in anatomy, rarely in medical terminology)
40. sinistro-	a. to the left b. left side
41. sub-	a. under b. below c. beneath d. in small quantity e. less than normal
42. super-	a. above average b. beyond the normal; to an especially high degree
43. supra-	a. above (a location or position)
44. syn- sym- (affixed to components beginning with b, p, m)	a. together
45. tachy-	a. rapid b. fast
46. trans-	a. across b. over

NUMBERS: PREFIXES

Prefix	*Meaning*
47. bi-	a. two b. twice c. double
48. di-	a. double b. twice c. two
49. tri-	a. three
50 quadri-	a. four
51. uni-	a. one

COLORS

Combining Form	*Meaning*
52. albo	white
53. chloro	green
54. chromo chromato	color
55. cyano	blue
56. erythro	red
57. melano	black
58. leuko	white leuco
59. polio	gray
60. rube	red rubri
61. xantho	yellow

Student Practice Activities

Activity 1

Flash Cards

Make prefix and color combining form flash cards. Make a separate card for each component. Print the correctly spelled prefix or combining form on one side of the card and the definition on the opposite side.

Activity 2

Memorize all components of this module.

Practice identifying/reciting/writing component definitions.

Practice identifying/reciting/writing correct component.

Activity 3

Word Building and Defining

The following activity demonstrates how the addition of a prefix qualifies the meaning of a medical term. The noun suffix used in the three (3) examples is –cardia. Using the rules of Module 3 – combine the following components to form a word.

Note: the changing of a prefix modifies the word meaning but does not change the meaning of the word.

Prefix	Noun Suffix	Medical Term & Definition
Example:		
a. tachy– (rapid, fast)	–cardia (heart)	tachycardia (rapid heart beat)
b. brady– (slow)	–cardia (heart)	bradycardia (slow heart beat)
c. dextro– (to the right)	–cardia (heart)	dextrocardia (heart on right side of body)

Prefix	Noun Suffix	Medical Term Formed	Definition
1. bi–	–lateral		
2. tri–	–lateral		
3. quadri–	–lateral		
4. dys–	–pepsia		
5. eu–	–pepsia		
6. a–, an–	–phasia		
7. hyper–	–phagia		
8. uni–	–cellular (cell)		
9. retro–	–cardia		
10. hemi–	–plegia		
11. eu–	–phonia		

Activity 3

Word Building and Defining (continued)

Prefix	Noun Suffix	Medical Term Formed	Definition
12. dys–	–phagia		
13. poly–	–dipsia		
14. oligo–	–pnea		
15. a–, an–	–uria		
16. dys–	–phasia		
17. intra–	–cellular		
18. inter–	–cellular		
19. hyper–	–pnea		
20. hypo–	–pnea		
21. eu–	–sthenia		
22. hyper–	–kinesis (movement, motion)		
23. brady–	–kinesis		
24. tachy–	–kinesis		
25. anti–	–emesis		
26. neo–	–plasm		
27. macro–	–glossia (tongue)		
28. supra–	–nasal (pertaining to the nose)		
29. trans–	–dermal (pertaining to skin)		
30. post–	–nasal (pertaining to the nose)		

Color/Prefix Crossword Puzzle

Activity 4

Complete prefix crossword puzzle using clues provided. All components are prefixes—root stems or word roots, from this module. There are no repeat components.

ACROSS		DOWN	
1. located under, below	27. slow	2. not, without	22. all, total
2. against	29. painful, difficult	4. opposite	28. twice, double
3. large	31. self	5. with, together	30. left side
5. in association (b,m,p)	33. half (partial)	6. white	31. away from
6. side	35. behind, in back of	7. three	32. outside, external
8. same	38. small	8. half, lateral	34. red
9. before	39. absent, without	11. out of, away from	36. upon
10. white	41. two	12. within, inside	37. straight
(variation of #6 Down)	42. between	14. under	40. located above
13. married ladies title	44. good, normal	15. black	43. after, behind
15. author's name	45. red	16. within, inside	45. red (root stem)
16. within	46. fast	17. false	49. before, forward
17. around	47. together, with	18. outside, in addition to	51. grey
20. blue	48. above, excessive	19. many, much	54. yellow
21. across	50. less than, decrease	20. color (anatomic root)	55. above average
23. right	52. few, scant		56. to, toward
24. one	53. green		
25. beside, beyond	57. four		
26. white (root stem)	58. new		

Medical Terminology – Color/Prefix Crossword Puzzle

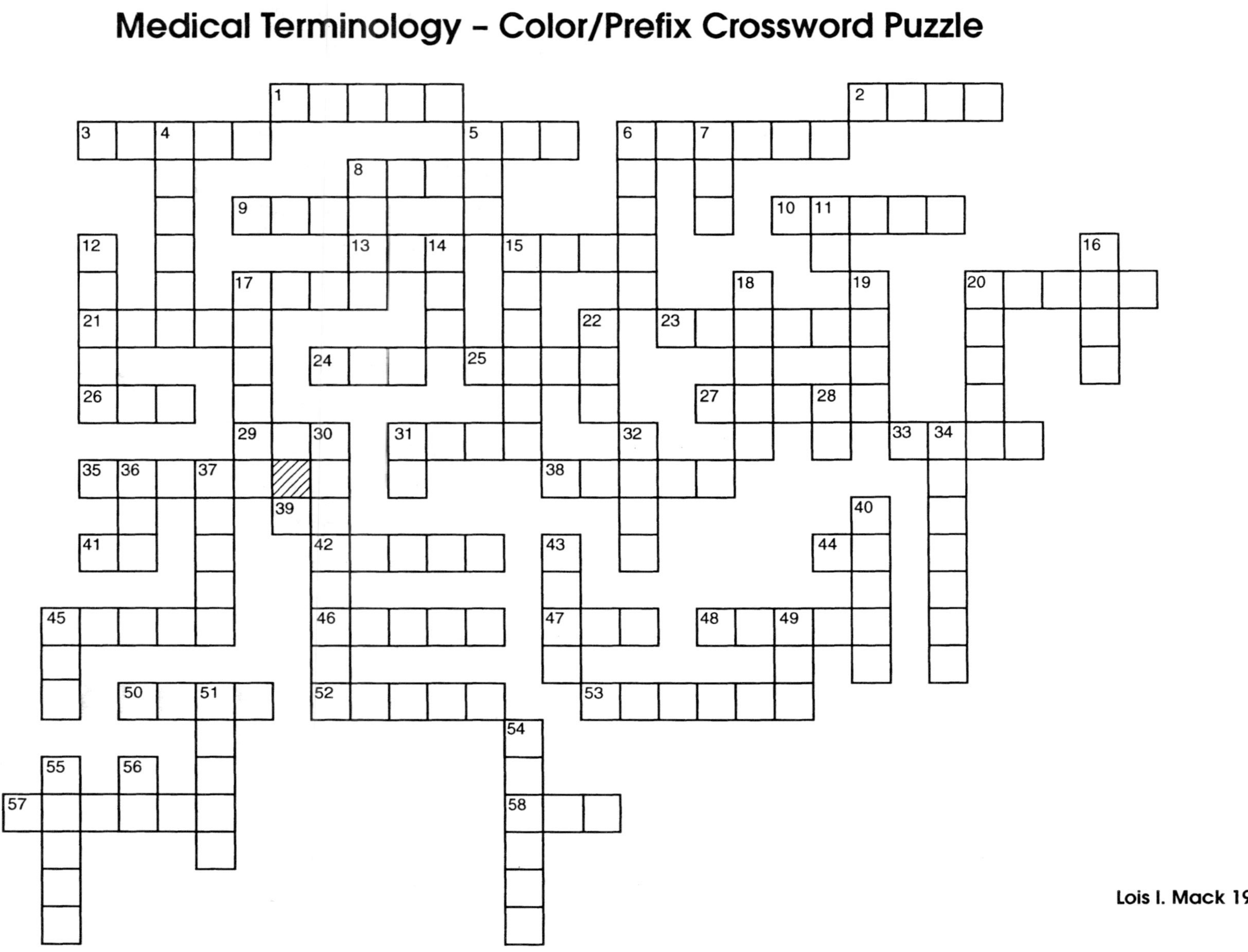

Solutions to Activities – Prefixes

Activity 3

Word Building and Defining

1. bilateral — pertaining to both sides
2. trilateral — pertaining to three sides
3. quadrilateral — pertaining to four sides
4. dyspepsia — painful digestion, difficulty with digestion, indigestion is commonly used term
5. eupepsia — normal digestion, good digestion
6. aphasia — no speech; inability to form language
7. hyperphagia — excessive eating
8. unicellular — having one cell
9. retrocardia — behind the heart
10. hemiplegia — paralysis on one half of body—left or right side
11. euphonia — normal speech, normal voice
12. dysphagia — difficulty swallowing, painful swallowing
13. polydipsia — much thirst, excessive thirst
14. oligopnea — infrequent breathing, very slow breathing
15. anuria — no urine being formed
16. dysphasia — difficulty forming words, difficulty communicating with words
17. intracellular — pertaining to within cell(s)
18. intercellular — pertaining to between cell(s)
19. hyperpnea — over-breathing, excessive breathing, hyperventilation

Activity 3

Word Building and Defining (continued)

20.	hypopnea	shallow breathing, decrease depth and rate of respiration
21.	eusthenia	normal strength
22.	hyperkinesis	excessive movement
23.	bradykinesis	slow movement
24.	tachykinesis	rapid movement
25.	antiemesis	against vomiting, to prevent vomiting
26.	neoplasm	new tissue formation
27.	macroglossia	enlarged tongue
28.	supranasal	pertaining to above the nose
29.	transdermal	pertaining to across or through the skin
30.	postnasal	pertaining to after or behind the nose

Solutions to Activities – Prefixes

Prefixes Crossword Puzzle

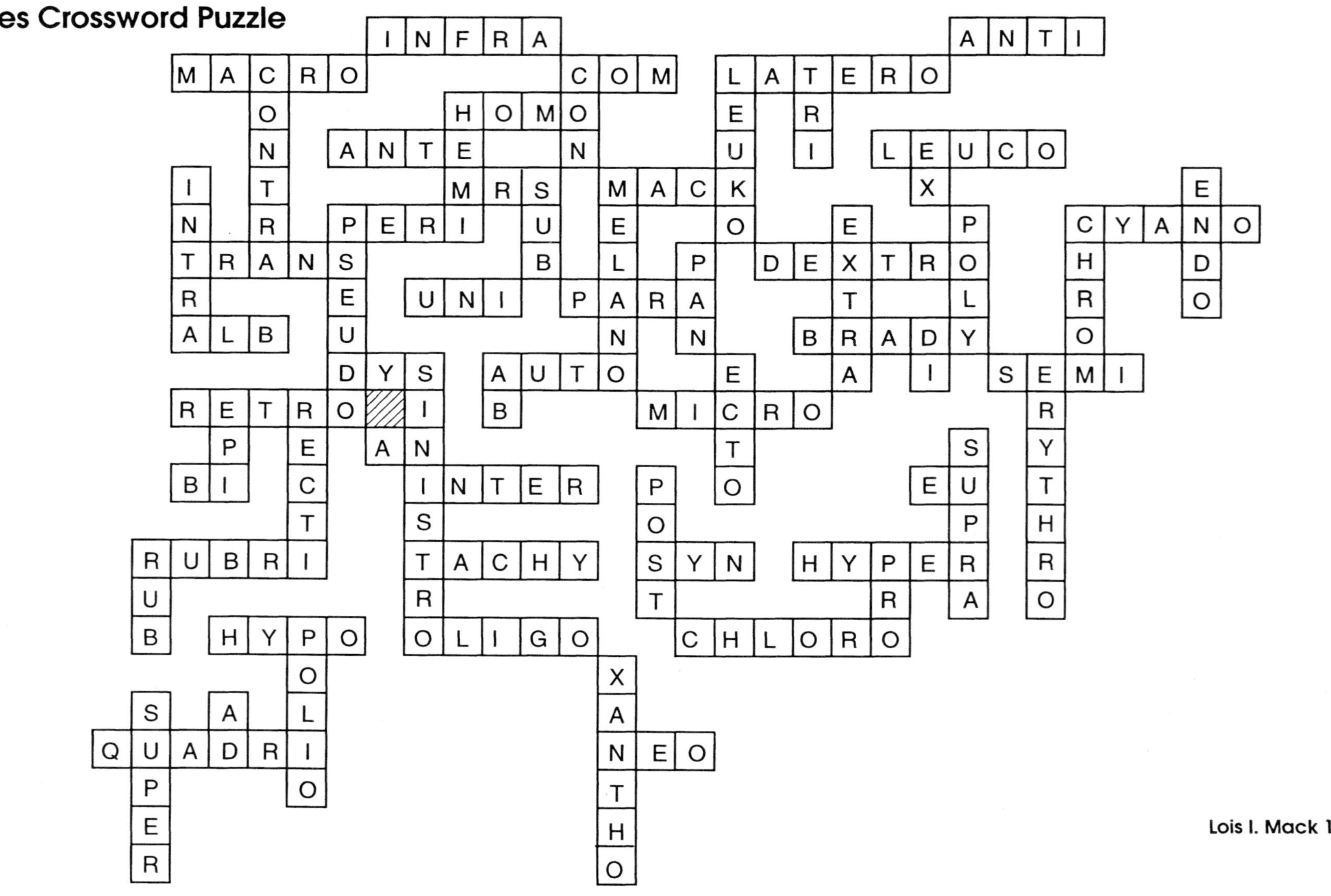

Lois I. Mack 1996

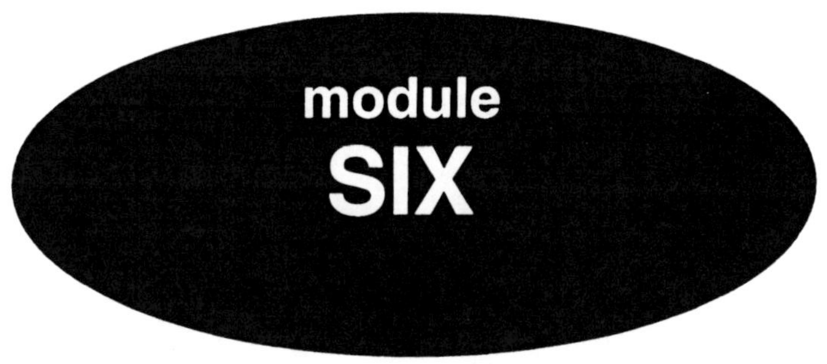

Musculoskeletal System

Objectives

Upon completion of these modules the student should be able to:

1. Identify and differentiate prefixes, suffixes, root stems and combining forms of this unit.

2. Write the correctly spelled component, given a list of definitions.

3. Write the definitions for each, given a list of components.

4. Divide the medical term(s) into individual appropriate components; using these definitions, construct a sentence to define the word.

5. Assign the appropriate components to build a medical term when given a medical sentence and construct a correctly spelled medical term.

6. Complete all activities in each module correctly.

The Musculoskeletal System

A. Structure and Functions

The Musculoskeletal System includes all bones, joints, muscles, tendons, cartilage and ligaments of the body. This system is responsible for providing body support and shape; protection for internal organs; mobility or movement; storage of calcium; and hemopoiesis. The human skeleton is made up of 206 bones. There are hundreds of muscles in the human body. Structures of the Musculoskeletal System are composed of connective tissue.

B. Components Pertaining to the Skeletal System

Combining Form	Meaning
1. arthro	joint
2. burso	bursa (bursae–pl.)
3. carpo	wrist (bones of)
4. cephalo	head
5. chondro	cartilage: gristle
6. claviculo cleido	clavicle: collar bone
7. costo	ribs
8. cranio	cranium: skull
9. dactylo	fingers/toes: digits
10. diaphysio diaphyseo	diaphysis: shaft of long bone
11. endosteo	endosteum: lining of the bone
12. epiphysio epiphyseo	epiphysis: growth end of long bone

Combining Form	*Meaning*
13. femoro	femur: thigh bone
14. fibulo	fibula: small bone of lower leg
15. tibio	tibia: shin bone of lower leg
16. humero	humerus: bone of upper arm
17. myelo	bone marrow
18. osteo	bone
19. periosteo	periosteum: membrane covering bone
20. phalango	bones of fingers/toes
21. rachio	spinal column: backbone
22. radio	radius: large long bone on thumb side of the forearm
23. spino	spine: any bone projection
24. spondylo	vertebra, (vertebrae–pl): individual bones of spinal column
25. synovio	synovial membrane/fluid
26. ulno	ulna: smaller long bone on the little finger side of the forearm
27. vertebro	vertebra: individual bones of the spinal column. Used in anatomical location, and not used for medical terms

C. Components Pertaining to the Muscular System and to Connective Tissues

Combining Form	*Meaning*
1. fascio	fascia: connective tissue that covers muscle or connects the skin to the underlying tissue
2. leiomyo	smooth muscle: involuntary muscles, muscles of the *viscera:* internal organs
3. ligamento	ligament: connective tissue which connects bone to bone. This form usually used for anatomical descriptions.
4. myo	muscle: meat of body myoso

Combining Form	*Meaning*
5. rhabdomyo	striated muscle: voluntary muscle, skeletal muscle
6. syndesmo	ligament: this component usually used in medical terminology
7. tendino tendo tendono teno	tendon: connective tissue which connects bone to muscle

D. Additional Components

Combining Form	*Meaning*
1. acro–	*extremity, appendage*
2. –clasis	surgical fracture
3. –poiesis	formation of, manufacturing of
4. –porosis	porous, lessened in density
5. –tonos, –tonia	muscle tone, muscle elasticity
6. –kinesis, –kinesia (*kinesis*)	body muscle, movement, motion
7. –cyte(s)	cell(s)
8. –pyo	pus
9. thoraco, –thorax (noun suffix)	chest

NOTE: Italicized words defined in Vocabulary.

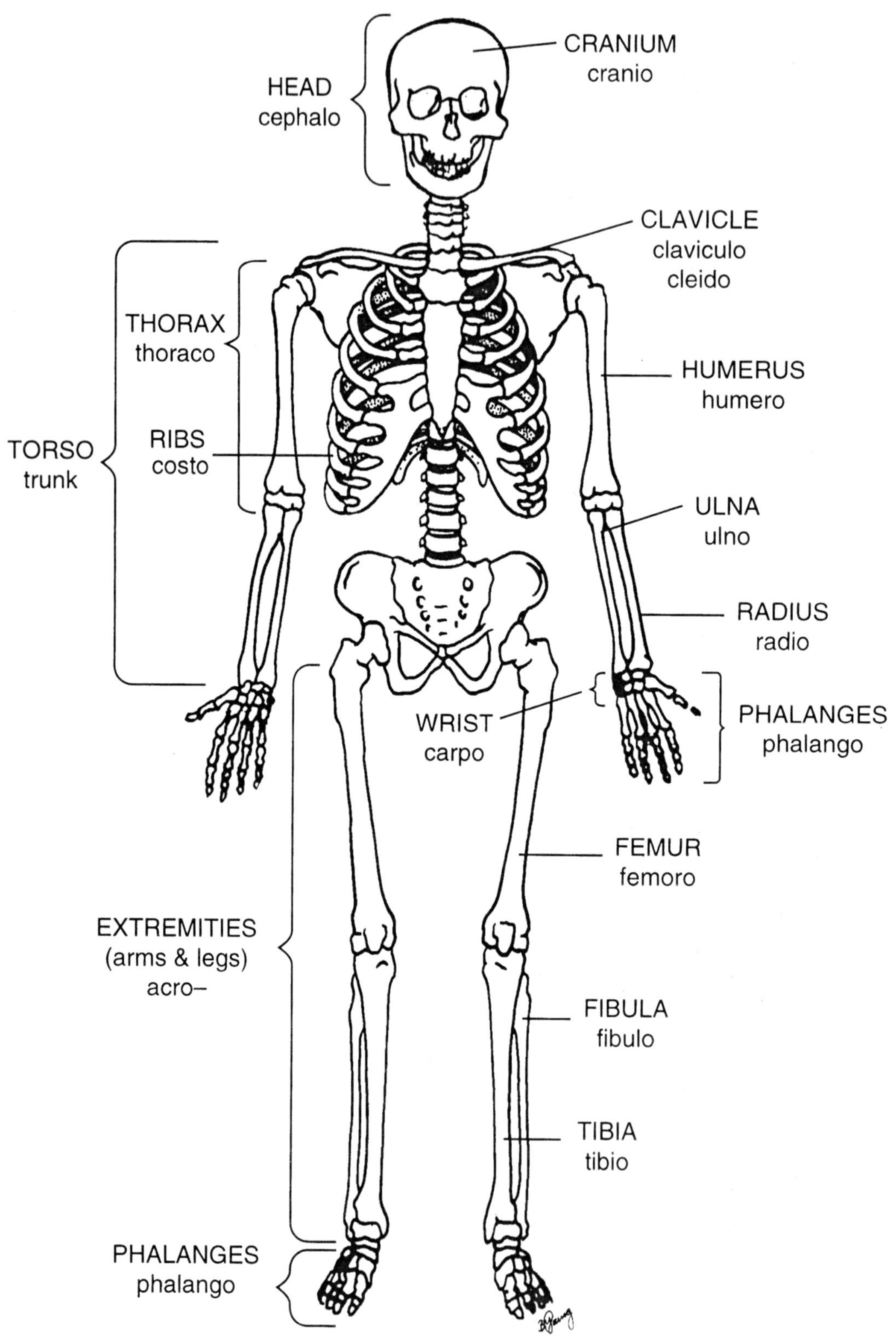

Figure 5.1. Major Bones of Skeletal System

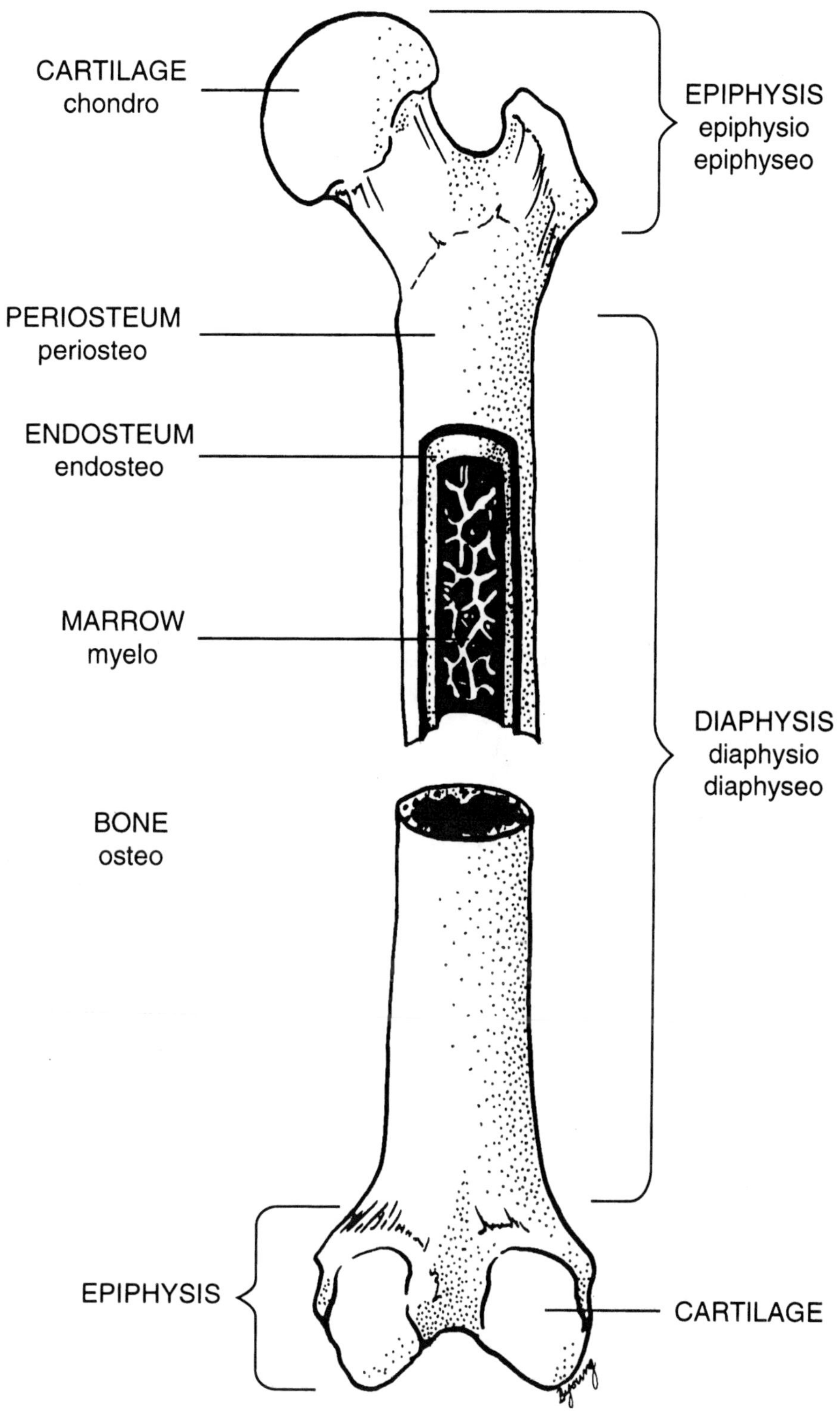

Figure 5.2. Structures of a Long Bone

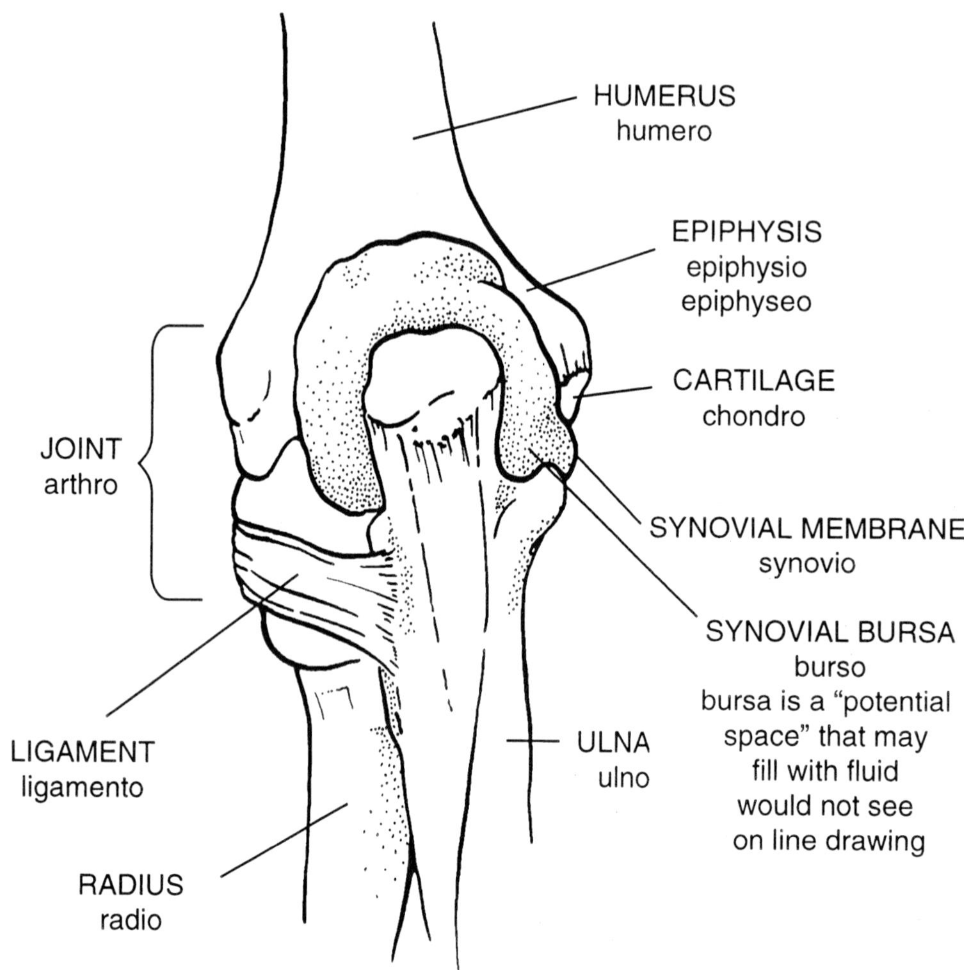

Figure 5.3. Dorsal View of the Elbow Joint

Student Practice Activities – Musculoskeletal System

Activity 1

Flash Cards

Make flash cards. Print the correctly spelled component on one side of the index card and the definition on the opposite side. Make additional flash cards for new components located on diagrams.

Activity 2

Figures 5.1–3. Study figures 5.1–3 in this module to become familiar with anatomy and related new components.

Activity 3

Memorize all new components pertaining to the Musculoskeletal System. All components must be spelled correctly.

Activity 4

Review Suffixes

Use flash cards to review *Suffixes*. Suffixes must be correctly spelled.

Activity 5

Review Prefixes

Use flash cards to review *Prefixes*. Prefixes must be correctly spelled.

Activity 6

Word Analysis: Combining Forms and Suffixes

Look at each medical term, determine the number of components in the word. Identify the requested components. Do not define components.

Medical Term	No. Components	Root Stem/Combining Form	Suffix
Example: arthritis	(2)	arthro	–itis
1. arthroma	( )		
2. arthrotherapy	( )		
3. arthrectomy	( )		
4. arthrosis	( )		
5. arthralgia	( )		
6. arthrodynia	( )		
7. spondylitis	( )		
8. spondylodesis	( )		
9. spondyloplasty	( )		
10. spondylotomy	( )		
11. rachiodynia	( )		
12. rachiomalacia	( )		
13. rachiopathy	( )		
14. rachiocentesis	( )		
15. rachiosarcoma	( )		

Activity 6

Word Analysis: Combining Forms and Suffixes (continued)

Medical Term	No. Components	Root Stem/Combining Form	Suffix
16. myorrhexis	( )		
17. myopathy	( )		
18. myosalgia	( )		
19. myosorrhaphy	( )		
20. myosorrhexis	( )		
21. chondromegalia	( )		
22. chondrogenic	( )		
23. chondrectomy	( )		
24. chondroid	( )		
25. tendinotomy	( )		
26. tendinodynia	( )		
27. tendodesis	( )		
28. osteochondritis	( )		
29. osteomyelocentesis	( )		
30. chondromyoma	( )		
31. chondroarthroscopy	( )		
32. osteoarthrosarcoma	( )		
33. rhabdomyospasm	( )		
34. leiomyorrhage	( )		
35. chondromalacia	( )		

Activity 6

Combining Components to Form Words: Prefixes + Combining Forms + Suffixes

Divide the following medical terms into components. Identify the components by recording them in the appropriate blanks. Do not define components.

Medical Term	No. Components	Prefix	Combining Form(s) Root Stem(s)	Suffix
Example:				
pan/myo/lysis	(3)	pan-	myo	-lysis
intra/cranium	(2)	intra-		-cranium (noun suffix)
1. bradykinesis	( )			
2. polyosteoclasis	( )			
3. dyssyndesmospasm	( )			
4. arthropyosis (pyo=pus)	( )			
5. intercostal	( )			
6. hemiparesis	( )			
7. polydactylism	( )			
8. trilateral	( )			
9. extraspinal	( )			
10. microcephalic	( )			

Activity 7

Combining Components – Word Formation

1. Review rules of combining (Module 2) before beginning this exercise.
2. Join the components in each problem to form a correctly spelled word.
3. Do not define the word formed.
4. Remember to apply rules for the use of combining vowels.

Correctly Spelled Medical Term

Example:

arthro	–itis	arthritis
1. periosteo	–lysis	
2. syndesmo	–plasty	
3. sydesm	–sarcoma	
4. syndesmo	–oma	
5. tend	–rrhaphy	
6. tendino	–ectomy	
7. tendino	–plasty	
8. osteo	–penia	
9. osteo	–clasis	
10. osteo	–graphy	
11. osteo	–sarcoma	
12. arthr	–ology	
13. arthro	–ectomy	
14. arthro	–malacia	

Activity 7

Combining Components – Word Formation (continued)

Correctly Spelled Medical Term

15. arthr   -genic
16. pan-   rachio   -plasty
17. arthro   -centesis
18. syndesmo   -rrhexis
19. intra-   osteo   -itis
20. poly-   myoso   -rrhexis
21. fascio   -ectomy
22. claviculo   -clasis
23. latero-   fibulo   -lysis
24. trans-   diaphragmo   -cele
25. cranio   -otomy

Activity 8

Word Analysis for Definition

Define the following medical terms.

1. Read the medical term carefully.
2. Divide the term into components.
3. Write the number of components within the parentheses.
4. Using the definition of each component within the word write a *brief* definition in the appropriate blank.

Medical Term	Divided Term	No. Components	Definition
Example:			
osteodynia	osteo/dynia	(2)	pain in bone(s)
osteomalacia	osteo/malacia	(2)	softening of bone(s)
1. panosteosarcoma		( )	
2. osteectomy		( )	
3. osteogenic		( )	
4. ostealgia		( )	
5. osteitis		( )	
6. panarthritis		( )	
7. arthrectomy		( )	
8. intraarthroplasty		( )	
9. periarthralgia		( )	
10. hemimyoplegia		( )	

Activity 8

Word Analysis for Definition (continued)

Medical Term	Divided Term	No. Components	Definition
11. amyosthenia		( )	
12. amyotonia		( )	
13. myopathy		( )	
14. myalgia		( )	
15. myorrhexis		( )	
16. chondritis		( )	
17. chondrolysis		( )	
18. chondrorrhaphy		( )	
19. osteochondroporosis		( )	
20. oligochondromyocytes		( )	
21. osteomyelitis		( )	
22. rhabdomyosarcoma		( )	
23. leiomyoma		( )	
24. osteoarthrolysis		( )	
25. rhabdomyoparesis		( )	
26. tendinotomy		( )	
27. myesthesia		( )	
28. bursoarthrosis		( )	
29. periosteolysis		( )	
30. syndesmorrhaphy		( )	

Activity 9

Word Synthesis/Word Building

Follow instruction for word synthesis:

1. read sentence carefully.
2. select components necessary to build the word.
3. place components in the proper order for combining.
4. use the "Rules of Combining" to correctly join the components.

1. muscle spasm ____
2. plastic repair of cartilage and a joint _______________________________
3. surgical removal of a digit (finger or toe) ___________________________
4. tapping a joint for pus drainage ____________________________________
5. surgical reconstruction of the cranium ______________________________
6. a binding fixation of the spinal column _____________________________
7. a malignant tumor of the bone(s) ___________________________________
8. suspension of tendons ____
9. any disease of the extremities ______________________________________
10. rupture of the cartilage of the wrist ________________________________
11. enlarged head ____
12. resembling bone ____
13. tracing made of the electrical activity of muscles ____________________
14. more or less permanent opening of the cranium ______________________
15. manufacturing of, formation of bone marrow ________________________

Solutions to Practice Activity – Musculoskeletal System

Activity 6

Word Analysis – Combining Form(s)/Root Stem(s) + Suffix

Number of Components	Combining Form(s) Root Stem(s)	Suffix
(2)	arthr	-itis
1. (2)	arthr	-oma
2. (2)	arthro	-therapy
3. (2)	arthr	-ectomy
4. (2)	arthr	-osis
5. (2)	arthr	-algia
6. (2)	arthro	-dynia
7. (2)	spondyl	-itis
8. (2)	spondylo	-desis
9. (2)	spondylo	-plasty
10. (2)	spondyl	-otomy
11. (2)	rachio	-dynia
12. (2)	rachio	-malacia
13. (2)	rachio	-pathy
14. (2)	rachio	-centesis
15. (2)	rachio	-sarcoma
16. (2)	myo	-rrhexis

Activity 6

Word Analysis – Combining Form(s)/Root Stem(s) + Suffix (continued)

Number of Components	Combining Form(s) Root Stem(s)		Suffix
17. (2)		myo	-pathy
18. (2)		myos	-algia
19. (2)		myoso	-rrhaphy
20. (2)		myoso	-rrhexis
21. (2)		chondro	-megalia
22. (2)		chondro	-genic
23. (2)		chondr	-ectomy
24. (2)		chondr	-oid
25. (2)		tendin	-otomy
26. (2)		tendino	-dynia
27. (2)		tendo	-desis
28. (3)	osteo	chondr	-itis
29. (3)	osteo	myelo	-centesis
30. (3)	chondro	my	-oma
31. (3)	chondro	arthro	-scopy
32. (3)	osteo	arthro	-sarcoma
33. (2)		rhabdomyo	-spasm
34. (2)		leiomyo	-rrhage
35. (2)		chondro	-malacia

Activity 6

Combining Components to Form Words: Word Analysis – Prefix + Combining Form(s) + Suffix

Number of Components	Prefix	Combining Form(s) Root Stem(s)		Suffix
1. (2)	brady-			-kinesis
2. (3)	poly-	osteo		-clasis
3. (3)	dys-	syndesmo		-spasm
4. (3)		arthro	py	-osis
5. (3)	inter-	cost		-al
6. (2)	hemi-			-paresis
7. (3)	poly-	dactyl		-ism
8. (3)	tri-	later		-al
9. (3)	extra-	spin		-al
10. (3)	micro-	cephal		-ous

Activity 7

Combining Components

1.	periosteolysis	14.	arthromalacia
2.	syndesmoplasty	15.	arthrogenic
3.	syndesmosarcoma	16.	panrachioplasty
4.	syndesmoma	17.	arthrocentesis
5.	tendorrhaphy	18.	syndesmorrhexis
6.	tendonectomy	19.	intraosteitis
7.	tendinoplasty	20.	polymyosospasms
8.	osteopenia	21.	fasciectomy
9.	osteoclasis	22.	claviculoclasis
10.	osteography	23.	laterofibulolysis
11.	osteosarcoma	24.	transdiaphragmocele
12.	arthrology	25.	craniotomy
13.	arthrectomy		

Activity 8

Word Analysis for Definition

Divided Term	Number of Components	Definition
1. pan/osteo/sarcoma	(3)	malignancy of all the bone(s)
2. oste/ectomy	(2)	excision of bone(s)
3. osteo/genic	(2)	originating in bone(s)

Activity 8

Word Analysis for Definition (continued)

Divided Term	Number of Components	Definition
4. oste/algia	(2)	bone pain
5. oste/itis	(2)	inflammation of bone(s)
6. pan/arthr/itis	(3)	inflammation of all joints
7. arthr/ectomy	(2)	surgical removal of joint
8. intra/arthro/plasty	(3)	plastic repair within a joint
9. peri/arthr/algia	(3)	pain around the joint(s)
10. hemi/myo/plegia	(3)	paralysis of muscles on one side of body
11. a/myo/sthenia	(3)	no muscle strength
12. a/myo/tonia	(3)	no muscle tone
13. myo/pathy	(2)	any disease of muscle(s)
14. my/algia	(2)	muscle pain
15. myo/rrhexis	(2)	ruptured muscle
16. chondr/itis	(2)	inflamed cartilage
17. chondro/lysis	(2)	breakdown or freeing up of cartilage
18. chondro/rrhaphy	(2)	suturing of cartilage
19. osteo/chondro/porosis	(3)	lessened density of bone and cartilage
20. oligo/chondro/myo/cytes	(4)	a scant number of muscle and cartilage cells
21. osteo/myel/itis	(3)	inflamed bone and marrow; inflamed bone marrow
22. rhabdomyo/sarcoma	(2)	cancer of voluntary muscle(s)

Activity 8

Word Analysis for Definition (continued)

Divided Term	Number of Components	Definition
23. leiomy/oma	(2)	tumor of involuntary (smooth) muscle
24. osteo/arthro/lysis	(3)	breakdown of bone and joint
25. rhabdomyo/paresis	(2)	weakness of voluntary muscles
26. tendon/otomy	(2)	incision into tendon(s)
27. my/esthesia	(2)	perception of sensation or feeling of in muscle
28. burso/arthr/osis	(3)	abnormal condition of bursa and joint
29. periosteo/lysis	(2)	freeing up or breakdown of periosteum
30. syndesmo/rrhaphy	(2)	suturing of ligament

Activity 9

Word Synthesis/Word Building

1. myospasm, myosospasm
2. chondro-arthroplasty, arthrochondroplasty, chondroarthroplasty
3. dactylectomy, phalangectomy
4. pyoarthrocentesis, pyo-arthrocentesis, arthropyocentesis
5. cranioplasty
6. rachiodesis
7. osteosarcoma
8. tendinopexy, tendonopexy, tendopexy, tenopexy
9. acropathy
10. carpochondrorrhexis, chondrocarporrhexis
11. cephalomegalia, cephalomegaly
12. osteoid
13. electromyogram, electromyosogram
14. craniostomy
15. myelopoiesis

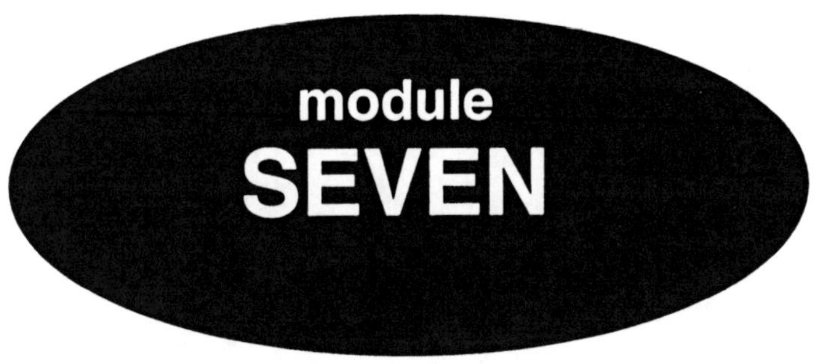

Respiratory System

Objectives

Upon completion of these modules the student should be able to:

1. Identify and differentiate prefixes, suffixes, root stems and combining forms of this unit.

2. Write the correctly spelled component, given a list of definitions.

3. Write the definitions for each, given a list of components.

4. Divide the medical term(s) into individual appropriate components; using these definitions, construct a sentence to define the word.

5. Assign the appropriate components to build a medical term when given a medical sentence and construct a correctly spelled medical term.

6. Complete all activities in each module correctly.

Respiratory System

A. Structure and Functions

The nose, nostrils, nasopharynx, pharynx (throat), larynx (vocal cords) and the lungs and the bronchi, bronchioles and alveoli form the major structures of this system. These structures form the external passageway for air to travel internally into the blood stream to supply the body cells with necessary oxygen. The respiratory system also functions to maintain the blood gas balance and assists with the heating/cooling functions of the body. The diaphragm is the muscular structure forming the floor of the thoracic cavity that assists the body to pull air into and to push it out of the lungs.

B. Components Pertaining to the Respiratory System

Combining Form	*Definition*
1. naso	nose
2. rhino	nose
3. nasopharyngo	passageway connecting the nose to the pharynx
4. sinuso	sinus
5. pharyngo	pharynx: throat
6. stomato	mouth, oral cavity
7. laryngo	larynx: vocal cords, voice box
8. tracheo	trachea: windpipe
9. thoraco thora (rare variation)	thorax: chest, chest cavity chest (used with –centesis only)

Combining Form	*Definition*
10. bronchio	bronchi and bronchioles: bronchial tree or tubes of the respiratory system
11. broncho	bronchus – sing., bronchi – pl.: large branches of respiratory tree
12. bronchiolo	bronchioles: small branches of respiratory tree
13. alveolo	alveolus, sing. (alveoli, pl.): air sacs of the lungs, *parenchyma*: functional tissue of lungs
14. pneumo	air when used with a noun suffix lung(s) when used with a regular suffix
15. pneumono, –pneumonon (noun suffix)	lung(s) only
16. pulmo pulmono, –pulmonon (noun suffix)	lung(s) only
17. mediastino	mediastinum: cavity between lungs containing the heart, its large vessels and the esophagus
18. pleuro	serosa: tissue lining closed round suffix cavities (pleura, sing.), (pleurae, pl.) pleural fluid; pleural cavity
19. lobo	lobes of an organ
20. thoraco thora –thorax	thorax: chest use only with –centesis present in the chest cavity

Additional Components*

Combining Form	*Definition*
21. atelo	incomplete formation or expansion of tissue
22. hemo, hemato	blood
23. hydro	fluid: any body fluid except blood or pus
24. litho, –lith(s),	stone(s), calculus (calculi, pl.)
25. pyo	pus
26. –atresia	absence of a normal body opening
27. –lithiasis	presence of stones, presence of calculus

Combining Form	*Definition*
28. –osmia, osmo	sense of smell, osmesis
29. –oxia	oxygen (usually in the blood stream)
30. –pnea	breath or breathing
31. –ptysis	spitting

*NOTE: Some of these components have appeared in Module 3.

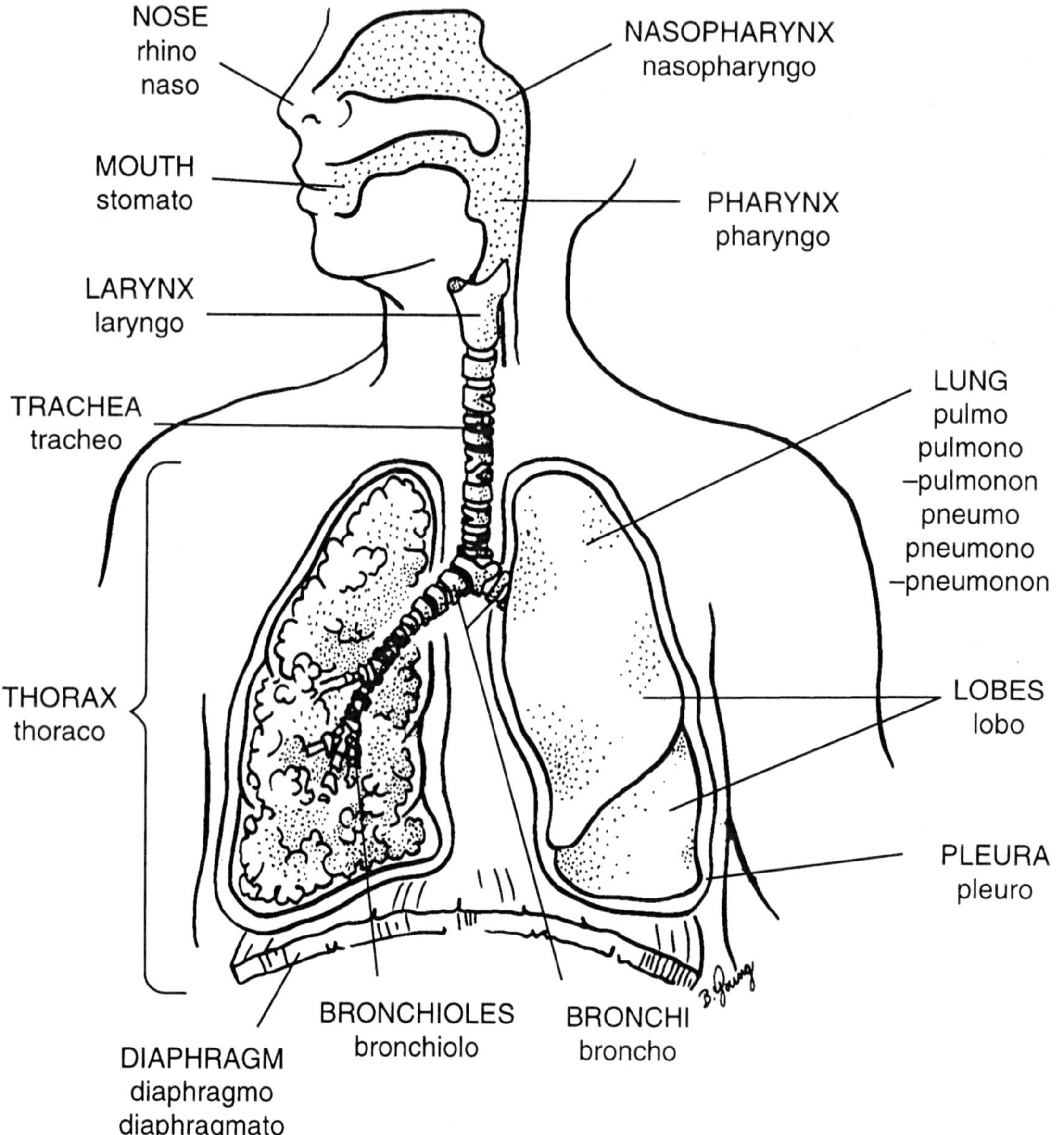

Figure 6.1. The Respiratory System

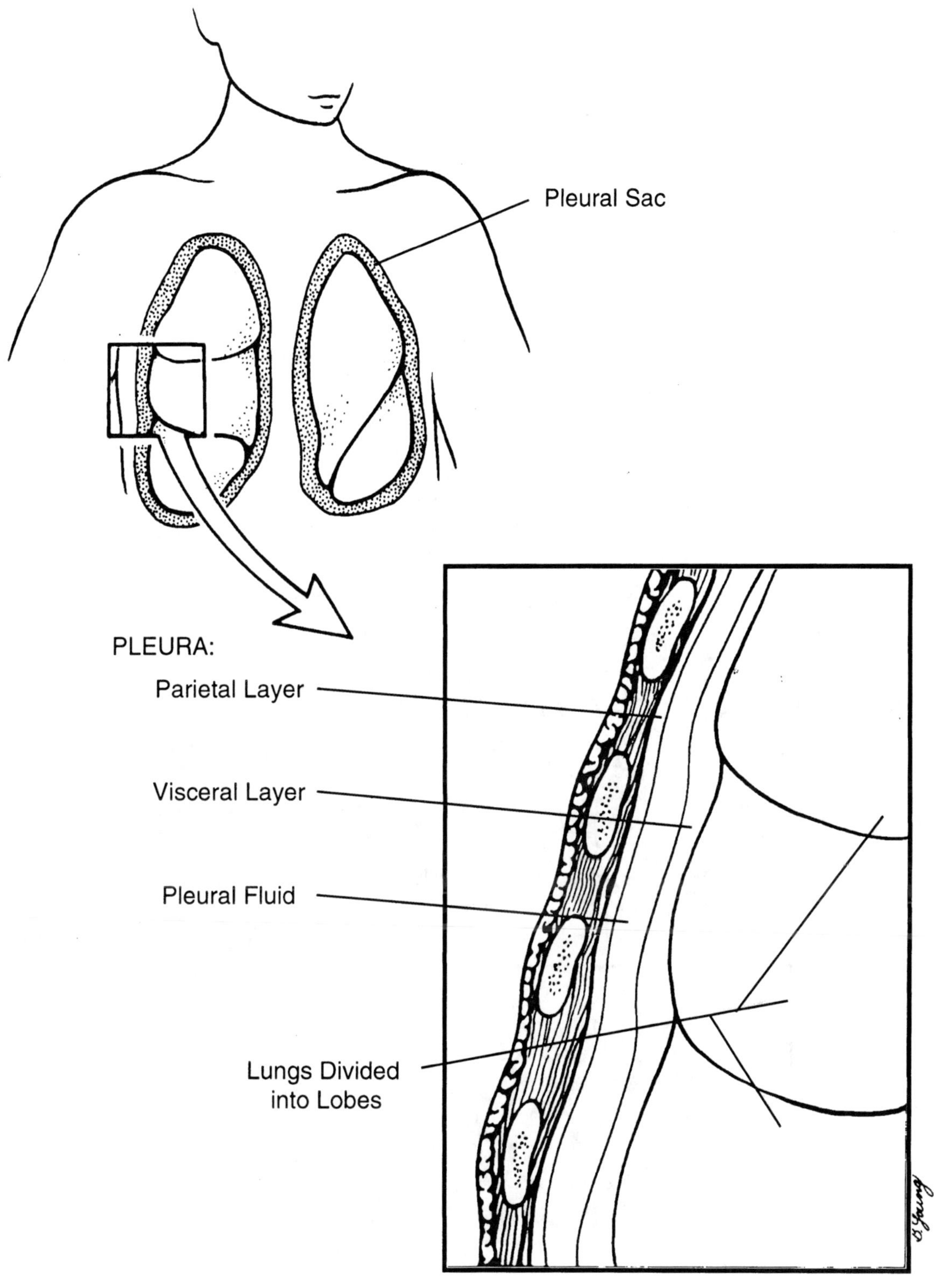

Figure 6.2. Structures of the Pleura

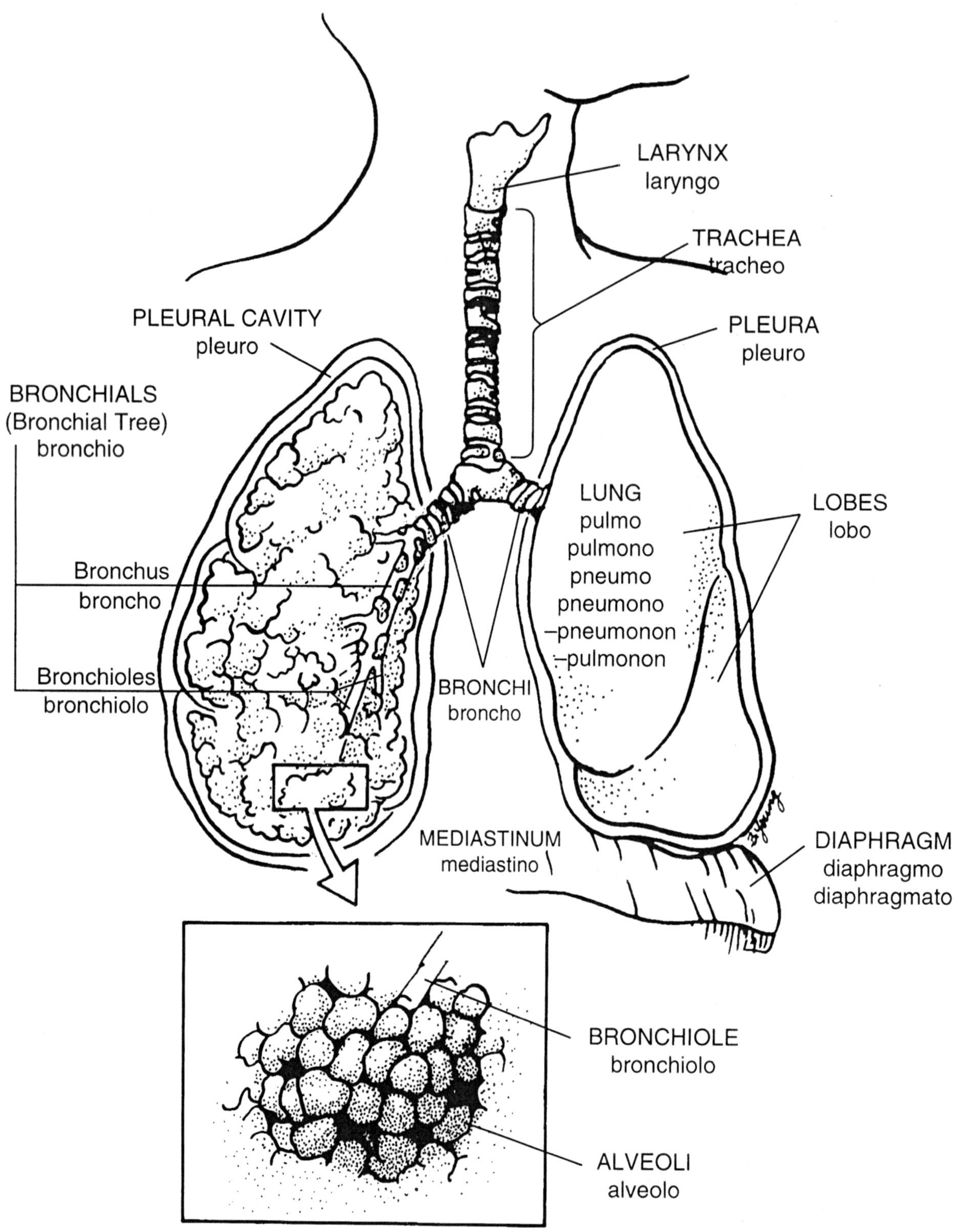

Figure 6.3. Structures for the Passage of Air in the Lungs

Student Activities – Respiratory System

Activity 1

Flash Cards

Make flash cards for this module, be sure to include components located on figures 6.1-3. Some components on list have been included. Check your flash cards for correct spelling.

Activity 2

Figures

Study figures (6.1-3) in this module for new components.

Activity 3

Memorize the new components and their definitions.

Activity 4

Review all suffixes and prefixes from previous modules. Practice reciting/writing definition when reviewing components. Practice reciting/writing components when looking at definitions.

Activity 5

Word Analysis

Look at each medical term and determine the number of components in that word. Identify and record each component in the correct column. Do not define components.

Medical Term	No. Components	Combining Form(s) Root Stem(s)	Suffix
Examples:			
rhino/rrhea	(2)	rhino	–rrhea
rhin/algia	(2)	rhin	–algia
1. rhinorrhagia	( )		
2. rhinogenic	( )		
3. rhinoclasis	( )		
4. rhinoliths	( )		
5. rhinolithiasis	( )		
6. pleurodynia	( )		
7. rhinolithotomy	( )		
8. panlaryngoplasty	( )		
9. perilaryngodynia	( )		
10. laryngostomy	( )		
11. bronchospasm	( )		
12. bronchitis	( )		
13. bronchiectasis	( )		

Activity 5

Word Analysis (continued)

Medical Term	No.	Components	Combining Form(s) Root Stem(s)	Suffix
14. bronchiospasm	( )			
15. pneumonectomy	( )			
16. thoracentesis	( )			
17. thoracostomy	( )			
18. thoracoplasty	( )			
19. tracheorrhagia	( )			
20. tracheostenosis	( )			
21. hemipharyngalgia	( )			
22. tracheoplasty	( )			
23. antibronchiolospasm	( )			
24. bronchiolectasis	( )			
25. pneumocele	( )			
26. pyoptysis	( )			
27. pyopneumonothorax	( )			
28. pleuralgia	( )			
29. pneumohydrothorax	( )			
30. hemohydropleura	( )			

Activity 6

Combining Components to Form Words

1. Review rules of combining (Module 2) before beginning this exercise.
2. Join the components in each problem to form a correctly spelled word.
3. Do not define the word formed.
4. Remember to apply rules for the use of combining vowels.

Prefix	Combining Forms	Suffix	
Example:			
	rhino	–pathy	rhinopathy
pan–	bronchio	–ectasis	panbronchiectasis
1.	laryngo	–spasm	
2.	broncho	–itis	
3.	pneumo	–thorax	
4.	pneumono	–ectomy	
5. tracheo	bronchio	–gram	
6.	bronch	–spasm	
7. pyo	pneumo	–pleura	
8.	thoraco	–centesis	
9. endo–	bronchio	–itis	
10.	rhino	–liths	
11.	pulmo	–genic	
12.	tracheo	–ostomy	
13.	bronchio	–al	

Activity 6

Combining Components to Form Words (continued)

Prefix	Combining Forms	Suffix	
14.	pleuro	–ectomy	__________
15. naso	pharyngo	–graphy	__________
16.	hemo	–ptysis	__________
17. pan–	thoraco	–plasty	__________
18. hyper–		–pnea	__________
19.	rhino	–rrhagia	__________
20. hemi–	lobo	–ectomy	__________

Activity 7

Word Analysis for Definition

Define the following medical terms.

1. Read the medical term carefully.
2. Divide the term into components.
3. Write the number of components within the parentheses.
4. Using the definition of each component within the word write a *brief* definition in the appropriate blank.

Medical Term	No. Components	Definition
1. rhinorrhea	( )	__________
2. laryngodynia	( )	__________
3. bronchitis	( )	__________

Activity 7

Word Analysis for Definition (continued)

Medical Term	No. Components	Definition
4. bronchiectasis	( )	
5. tracheobronchioplegia	( )	
6. rhinorrhagia	( )	
7. bronchiolospasm	( )	
8. thoracalgia	( )	
9. pulmopathy	( )	
10. thoracic	( )	
11. laryngitis	( )	
12. tracheostomy	( )	
13. hemopyopleura	( )	
14. thoracentesis	( )	
15. tracheotomy	( )	
16. bronchogenic	( )	
17. pleuritis	( )	
18. thoracocentesis	( )	
19. pharyngoplasty	( )	
20. bronchogram	( )	
21. bronchiolectasis	( )	
22. pneumocele	( )	

Activity 7

Word Analysis for Definition (continued)

Medical Term	No. Components	Definition
23. sinusalgia	( )	
24. nasopharyngostomy	( )	
25. diaphragmatoplegia	( )	

Activity 8

Word Synthesis/Word Building from a Sentence

Follow instruction for word synthesis:

1. Read sentence carefully.
2. Select component necessary to build the word.
3. Place components in the proper order for combining.
4. Use the "Rule for Combining" to correctly join the components.

Example:

absence of the normal opening into the trachea

–atresia   tracheo

tracheoatresia; tracheatresia

1. dilatation of the bronchioles

Activity 8

Word Synthesis/Word Building from a Sentence (continued)

2. a breakdown of the lung tissue

3. narrowing of the trachea

4. pain in the throat

5. x-ray of the entire bronchial tree

6. flow of pus from the sinus

7. temporary opening of the chest

8. air in the chest

Activity 8

Word Synthesis/Word Building from a Sentence (continued)

9. blood in the lungs

10. pus and air in the pleural cavity

11. pus and blood in the lungs and pleura

12. uncontrolled contraction of the diaphragm

13. inflammation of larynx and throat

14. nasal hemorrhage

15. difficulty breathing

Solutions to Practice Activities – Respiratory System

Activity 5

Word Analysis

No.	Components	Prefix	Combining Form(s) Root Stem(s)	Suffix
	(2)		rhino	–rrhea
	(2)		rhin	–algia
1.	(2)		rhino	–rrhagia
2.	(2)		rhino	–genic
3.	(2)		rhino	–clasis
4.	(2)		rhino	–liths
5.	(2)		rhino	–lithiasis
6.	(2)		pleuro	–dynia
7.	(2)		rhino	–lithotomy
8.	(3)	pan–	laryngo	–plasty
9.	(3)	peri–	laryno	–dynia
10.	(2)		laryng	–ostomy
11.	(2)		broncho	–spasm
12.	(2)		bronch	–itis
13.	(2)		bronchi	–ectasis
14.	(2)		bronchio	–spasm
15.	(2)		pneumon	–ectomy

Activity 5

Word Analysis (continued)

No. Components	Prefix	Combining Form(s) Root Stem(s)	Suffix
16. (2)		thora	–centesis
17. (2)		thorac	–ostomy
18. (2)		thoraco	–plasty
19. (2)		tracheo	–rrhagia
20. (2)		tracheo	–stenosis
21. (3)	hemi–	pharyng	–algia
22. (2)		tracheo	–plasty
23. (3)	anti–	bronchiolo	–spasm
24. (2)		bronchiol	–ectasis
25. (2)		pneumo	–cele
26. (2)		pyo	–ptysis
27. (2)	pyo	pneumono	–thorax
28. (2)		pleur	–algia
29. (3)	pneumo	hydro	–thorax
30. (3)	hemo	hydro	–pleura

Activity 6

Combining Components to Form Words Solutions

1. laryngospasm
2. bronchitis
3. pneumothorax
4. pneumonectomy
5. tracheobronchiogram
   bronchiotracheogram
6. bronchospasm
7. pyopneumopleura
   pneumopyopleura
8. thoracocentesis
9. endobronchiitis
   endobronchitis
10. rhinoliths
11. pulmogenic
12. tracheostomy
13. bronchial
14. pleurectomy
15. nasopharyngography
16. hemoptysis
17. panthoracoplasty
18. hyperpnea
19. rhinorrhagia
20. hemilobectomy

Activity 7

Word Analysis for Definitions–Solutions

1. (2)   runny nose, watery discharge from the nose
2. (2)   pain in the vocal cords
3. (2)   inflammation of the bronchi
4. (2)   dilatation of the bronchials
5. (3)   paralysis of the trachea and bronchial tree
6. (2)   nose bleed
7. (2)   uncontrolled contractions of the bronchioles
8. (2)   chest pain, pain the the thorax
9. (2)   any disease of the lung(s)
10. (2)   pertaining to or concerning the thorax
11. (2)   inflammation of the vocal cords
12. (2)   more or less permanent opening of the trachea
13. (3)   blood and pus in the pleura
14. (2)   puncture for aspiration of the thorax
15. (2)   temporary opening of the trachea
16. (2)   originating in the bronchial tree
17. 2(2)   inflammation of the pleura
18. (2)   puncture for aspiration of the chest
19. (3)   surgical reconstruction of the pharynx
20. (2)   an x-ray of the bronchi

Activity 7

Word Analysis for Definitions–Solutions (continued)

21. (2)   dilatation of the bronchioles
22. (2)   herniatioon of the lung tissue
23. (2)   pain in the sinus
24. (3)   forming a communication between the nose and throat for continuous flow
25. (2)   paralysis of the diaphragm

Activity 8

Word Synthesis/Word Building from a Sentence Solution

1. dilatation of   bronchioles
   –ectasis   bronchiolo
            bronchiolectasis

2. breakdown   lungs
   –lysis   pneumo, pneumono, pulmo, pulmono
        pneumolysis, pneumonolysis,
            pulmolysis, pulmonolysis

3. narrowing of   trachea
   –stenosis   tracheo
            tracheostenosis

4. pain   throat
   –algia   pharyngo
   –dynia
        pharyngalgia, pharyngodynia

Activity 8

Word Synthesis/Word Building from a Sentence Solution (continued)

5. x-ray   entire   bronchial tree

    –gram   pan–   bronchio

    panbronchiogram

6. flow   pus   sinus

    –rrhea   pyo   sinuso

    sinusopyorrhea

7. temporary opening   chest

    –otomy   thoraco

    thoracotomy

8. air   chest

    pneumo   thorax

    pneumothorax

9. blood   lungs

    hemo, hemato   –pneumonon, –pulmonon

    hemopneumonon, hemopulmonon, hematopneumonon, hematopulmonon

10. pus   air   pleura

    pyo   pneumo   –pleura

    pyopneumopleura

Activity 8

Word Synthesis/Word Building from a Sentence Solution (continued)

11. pus   blood   lungs   pleura

     pyo   hemo   pneumono   –pleura

     pyohemopneumonopleura

12. uncontrolled contractions   diaphragm

     –spasm   diaphragmo

     diaphragmospasm

13. inflammation of   larynx   throat

     –itis   laryngo   pharyngo

     laryngopharyngitis

14. nose   hemorrhage

     rhino   –rrhagia

     rhinorrhagia

15. difficulty   breathing

     dys–   –pnea

     dyspnea

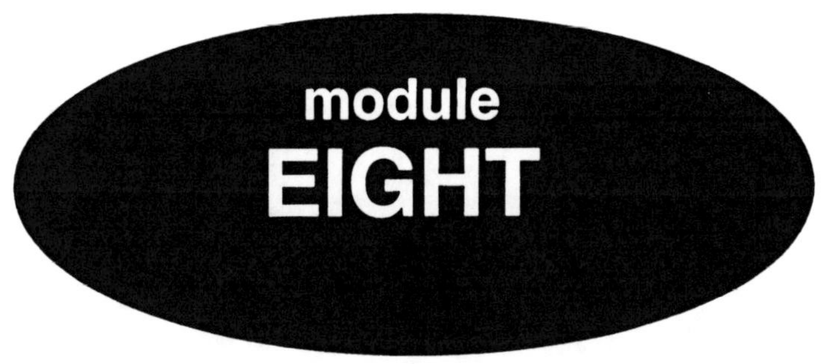

Digestive System

Objectives

Upon completion of these modules the student should be able to:

1. Identify and differentiate prefixes, suffixes, root stems and combining forms of this unit.

2. Write the correctly spelled component, given a list of definitions.

3. Write the definitions for each, given a list of components.

4. Divide the medical term(s) into individual appropriate components; using these definitions, construct a sentence to define the word.

5. Assign the appropriate components to build a medical term when given a medical sentence and construct a correctly spelled medical term.

6. Complete all activities in each module correctly.

The Digestive/Gastrointestinal/Alimentary System

A. Structures and Functions

The Digestive System is also called the Gastrointestinal System (G.I. System) or Alimentary System or Tract. Neither of the first two terms is quite accurate as descriptive terms. Digestive does not consider the elimination of waste products. Gastro-intestinal appears to begin the system in the stomach and does not consider structures preceding the stomach. Alimentary Tract would seem to be the most correct as it includes the activities of the entire system as well as the complete route including the accessory organs. The route includes the mouth and its structures, pharynx, esophagus, stomach, and intestines. The accessory organs include the salivary glands, liver, gallbladder, and the pancreas; these two groups of structures work together. They start and complete the functions of this system.

This system is concerned with the intake of foods; the route of foods through the body; the digestion and utilization of this intake; and elimination of the waste products.

B. Components Pertaining to the Alimentary System

NOTE: Components are listed in anatomical order as they occur in the passage of food from ingestion (taking in food) to elimination.

Combining Form	*Definition*
1. stomato	mouth, refers to oral mouth only
2. oro, ora	mouth, used to indicate the anatomical structure or pertaining to the mouth; not commonly used in forming medical words
3. cheilo	oral lips
4. labio	labia, any lip-like structure

Combining Form	*Definition*
5. glosso, –glossia	tongue
6. dento	teeth
7. gingivo	gingiva (gums)
8. bucco	cheeks
9. palato	hard palate (roof of the mouth)
10. tonsillo	tonsils
11. pharyngo	pharynx (throat)
12. esophago	esophagus
13. gastro	stomach
14. entero	intestines; general term for all intestines both small and large
15. duodeno	duodenum – first part of small intestine
16. jejuno	jejunum – second part of small intestine
17. ileo	ileum – third part of small intestine
18. colo	colon (large intestine)
colono	
19. ceco	cecum
20. appendico	appendix – used with any component
appendo	form usually used with –ectomy; rarely used with other suffixes
21. sigmoido	sigmoid colon
22. recto	rectum
23. ano	anus
24. procto	rectum and/or anus

Accessory Organs and Structures

25. sialo	saliva
26. sialangio	salivary duct
27. sialadeno	salivary gland
28. chole	bile, gall
29. cholangio	hepatic duct
30. cholecysto	gallbladder, cholecyst

Combining Form	*Definition*
31. choledocho	common bile duct
32. hepatico hepato	liver
33. pancreato pancreatico	pancreas

Additional Components

34. abdomino	abdomen
35. laparo	abdominal wall (flank)
36. viscero	*viscera*: internal organ enclosed within a cavity
37. –orexia	appetite
38. –anastomosis	a natural or surgical connection of two tubular structures
39. –ostomy	when used with two or more combining forms it means anastomosis
40. peritoneo	peritoneum: tissue which forms the serosa of the abdominal cavity.
41. lipo lipido	fat

Vocabulary for Module

1. appetite	a strong desire for satisfying a strong want or desire associated with pleasant sensations based on memories, usually for food.
2. bowels	the small and large intestines
3. cyst	fluid filled sac containing any fluid except blood or pus
4. edema	excessive increase of fluid in inter-cellular space of body tissues.
5. hunger	the uncomfortable sensation resulting from the lack of food
6. sphincter	circular muscle controlling a body orifice
7. stoma	a mouth-like opening, may be artificially created between a body cavity or passage to the outside, eg forming an outlet for the intestines on the abdominal wall.

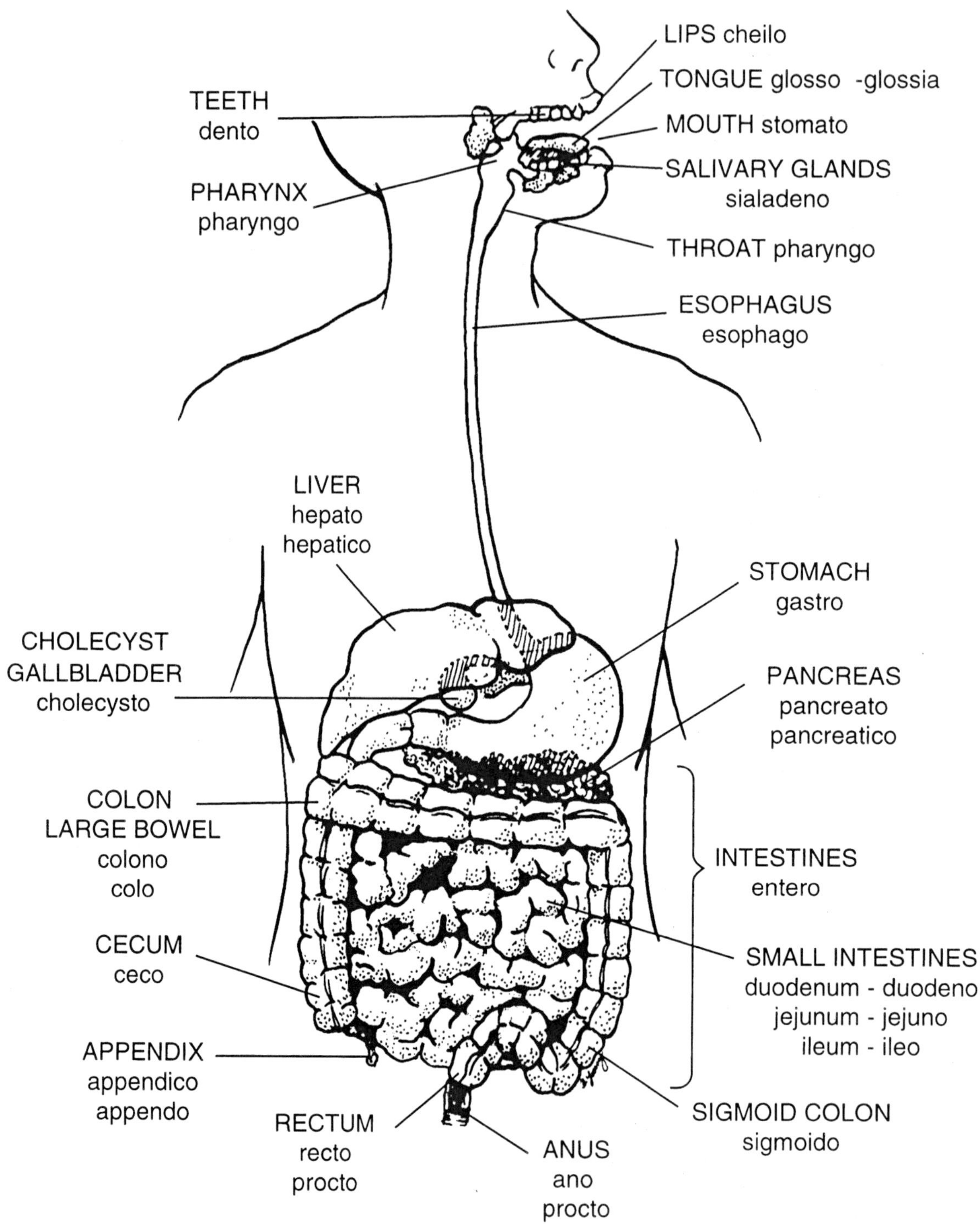

Figure 7.1. Digestive Tract and Accessory Organs

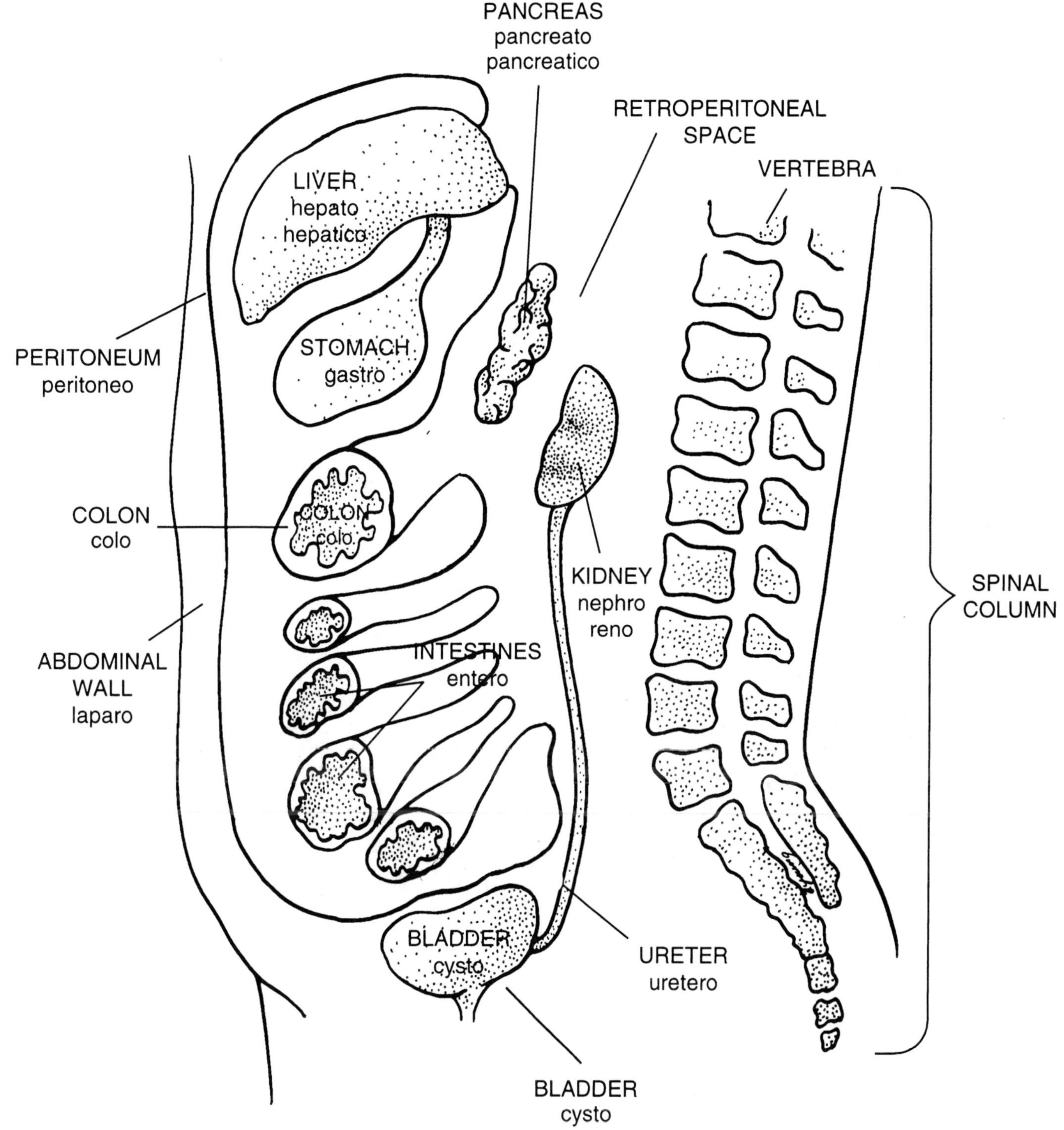

Figure 7.2. Lateral View of Peritoneal Cavity

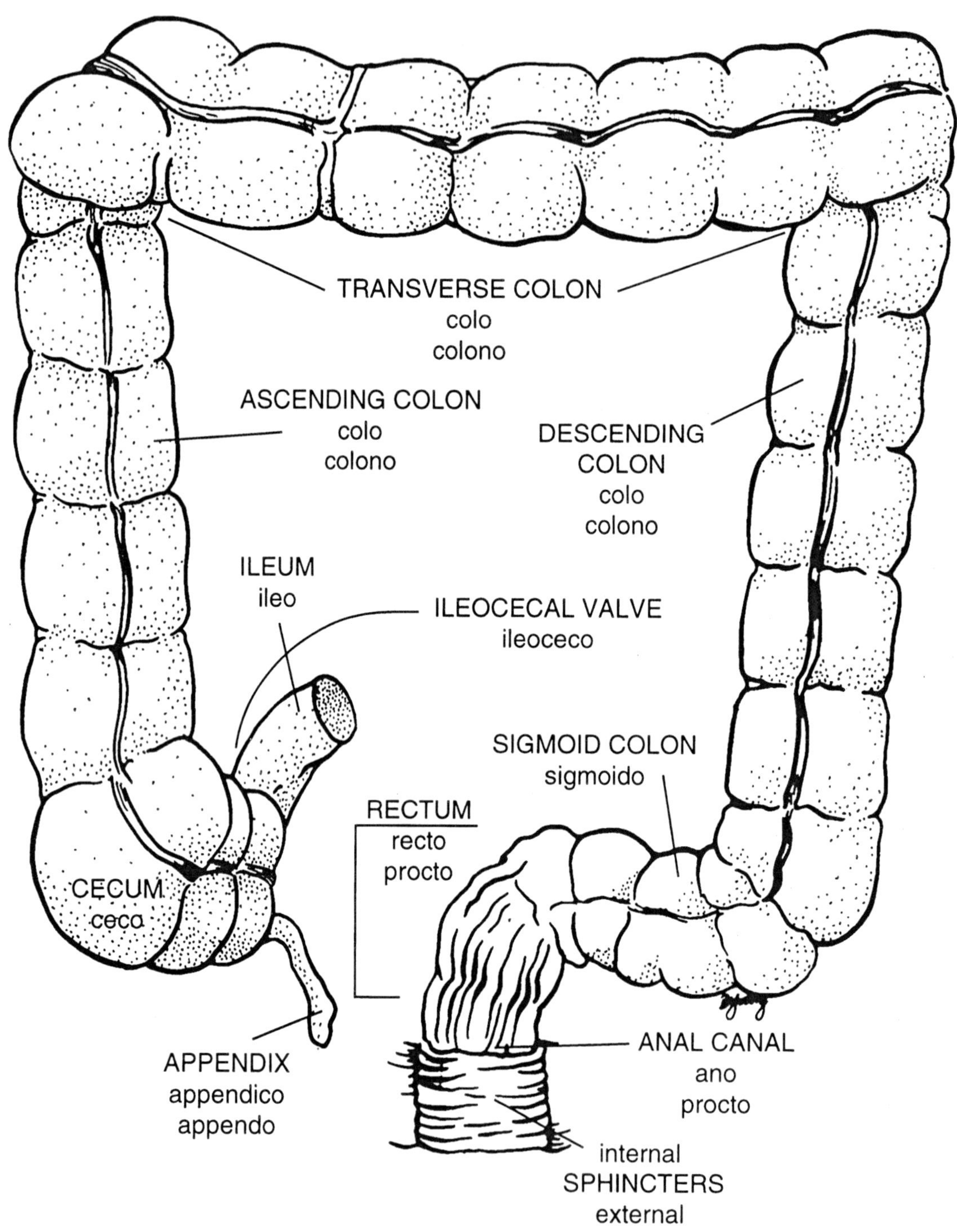

Figure 7.3. The Large Intestine

Student Practice Activities – Digestive System

Activity 1

Flash Cards

Make study cards by printing the new components on one side of the card and definitions on the opposite side. Include all new components from figures. Check for correct spelling. Add new words to Vocabulary Flash Cards.

Activity 2

Figures

Study Figures 7.1–3 in this module for new components. (Diagrams 7.1-3)

Activity 3

Memorize the new components and their definitions of this module.

Activity 4

Review all suffixes and prefixes from previous modules. Practice reciting/writing definition when reviewing the components. Practice reciting/writing components when looking at the definitions.

Activity 5

Word Analysis

Separate the following medical terms into components by placing each component in the proper column.

Medical Term	Number of Components	Prefix	Combining Form(s) Root Stems(s)	Suffix
Example: hemigastrectomy	(3)	hemi–	gastr	–ectomy
1. pharyngitis	( )			
2. gingivorrhaphy	( )			
3. peritonsillotomy	( )			
4. tonsillectomy	( )			
5. stomatoplasty	( )			
6. esophagectasis	( )			
7. esophagospasm	( )			
8. esophagorrhexis	( )			
9. gingivectomy	( )			
10. pharyngalgia	( )			
11. pharyngoplasty	( )			
12. enterostomy	( )			
13. enterorrhexis	( )			
14. duodenocele	( )			
15. enterocolocele	( )			
16. pancolomegalia	( )			

Activity 5

Word Analysis (continued)

Medical Term	Number of Components	Prefix	Combining Form(s) Root Stems(s)	Suffix
17. proctopexy	( )			
18. proctoscope	( )			
19. sigmoidoscopy	( )			
20. glossomegalia	( )			
21. euphagia	( )			
22. cholelithotomy	( )			
23. cholecystogram	( )			
24. cholangiolithiasis	( )			
25. gastroenterostomy	( )			
26. jejunostomy	( )			
27. cholelith	( )			
28. eupepsia	( )			
29. anosmia	( )			
30. peritonsillar	( )			
31. interdental	( )			

Activity 6

Defining Medical Terms

1. Read the medical term carefully
2. Divide the term into components
3. Write the number of components within the parentheses
4. Using the definition of each component within the term write a brief definition in the appropriate blank.

Medical Term	Divided Term	Number of Components	Definition
Example: subglossitis	sub/gloss/itis	(3)	inflammation under the tongue
1. dentodynia		( )	
2. pharyngostenosis		( )	
3. pharyngitis		( )	
4. labionasal		( )	
5. gingivitis		( )	
6. cheiloplasty		( )	
7. peritonsillotomy		( )	
8. tonsillectomy		( )	
9. endocolitis		( )	
10. stomatoplasty		( )	
11. esophagectasis		( )	
12. esophagorrhexis		( )	

Activity 6

Defining Medical Terms (continued)

Medical Term	Divided Term	Number of Components	Definition
13. sialorrhea		( )	
14. sialadenoedema		( )	
15. enterostomy		( )	
16. coloenterostomy		( )	
17. duodenocele		( )	
18. enteroplegia		( )	
19. pancolomegalia		( )	
20. proctoptosis		( )	
21. proctopexy		( )	
22. dyspepsia		( )	
23. dysosmia		( )	
24. cholecystogram		( )	
25. intradental		( )	
26. gastroileoanastomosis		( )	
27. cholecystolith(s)		( )	
28. cholecystolithiasis		( )	
29. cholecystolithotomy		( )	
30. sialadenosarcoma		( )	

Activity 6

Defining Medical Terms (continued)

Medical Term	Divided Term	Number of Components	Definition
31. pharyngalgia	__________________	( )	__________________
32. anorectoatresia	__________________	( )	__________________
33. proctoscopy	__________________	( )	__________________
34. pancreatorrhagia	__________________	( )	__________________
35. esophagoplegia	__________________	( )	__________________

Activity 7

Combine and Define

Join the components to form a properly spelled word. Define each word built; remember to define each component.

Prefix	Combining Form(s)	Suffix
Example:		
a–, an–	glosso	–ia

combine: aglossia
define: absence of a tongue

| 1. sub– | glosso | –itis |

combine: __________________

define: __________________

Activity 7

Combine and Define (continued)

Prefix	Combining Form(s)	Suffix
2. dento–		–dynia

combine: _______________________________

define: _______________________________

Prefix	Combining Form(s)	Suffix
3. intra–	tracheo	–rrhagia

combine: _______________________________

define: _______________________________

Prefix	Combining Form(s)	Suffix
4. entero		–spasm

combine: _______________________________

define: _______________________________

Prefix	Combining Form(s)	Suffix
5. stomato	esophago	–plasty

combine: _______________________ or _______________________

define: _______________________________

Prefix	Combining Form(s)	Suffix
6. peri–	tonsillo	–itis

combine: _______________________________

define: _______________________________

Activity 7

Combine and Define (continued)

Prefix	Combining Form(s)	Suffix
7. gingivo		–rrhea

combine: ____

define: ____

Prefix	Combining Form(s)	Suffix
8. dys–	gastro	–ia

combine: ____

define: ____

Prefix	Combining Form(s)	Suffix
9. chole		–centesis

combine: ____

define: ____

Prefix	Combining Form(s)	Suffix
10. a–, an–		–osmia

combine: ____

define: ____

Prefix	Combining Form(s)	Suffix
11. hyper–	gastro	–kinesia

combine: ____

define: ____

Activity 7

Combine and Define (continued)

Prefix	Combining Form(s)		Suffix
12. ano			–atresia
combine:			
define:			
13. pan–	duodeno	jejuno	–megalia
combine:			
define:			
14. colo			–ostomy
combine:			
define:			
15. gastro			–spasms
combine:			
define:			
16. hemi–	esophago		–plegia
combine:			
define:			

Activity 7

Combine and Define (continued)

Prefix	Combining Form(s)	Suffix
17. entero	entero	–ostomy

combine: _______________________ or _______________________

define: _______________________

| 18. hypo– | sialo | –rrhea |

combine: _______________________

define: _______________________

| 19. inter– | dento | –al |

combine: _______________________

define: _______________________

| 20. gastro | ileo | –anastomosis |

combine: _______________________ or _______________________

define: _______________________

| 21. esophago | | –stenosis |

combine: _______________________

define: _______________________

Activity 7

Combine and Define (continued)

Prefix	Combining Form(s)	Suffix
22. sialangio		–ectasis

combine: ____

define: ____

23. pharyngo		–dynia

combine: ____

define: ____

24. bucco	cheilo	–lysis

combine: ____

define: ____

25. hepato		–ectomy

combine: ____

define: ____

Activity 8

Word Synthesis/Word Building

1. Read sentence carefully.
2. Select components necessary to build the word.
3. Place components in the proper order for combining.
4. Use the "Rules of Combining" to correctly join the components.

Example:

narrowing of the trachea

components:	–stenosis	tracheo
order:	tracheo	–stenosis
term formed:	tracheostenosis	

1. toothache

2. plastic repair of the mouth and lips

3. hemorrhage of the pancreas

Activity 8

Word Synthesis/Word Building (continued)

4. normal voice

5. inflammation within the colon

6. feces harden like stones in colon

7. surgical removal of gallbladder

8. incision into the abdominal wall

Activity 8

Word Synthesis/Word Building (continued)

9. enlargement of the small and large intestines

10. surgical repair of the lip

11. stones of the salivary gland (already removed)

12. presence of stones in the gallbladder

13. anastomosis of the stomach to the duodenum

Activity 8

Word Synthesis/Word Building (continued)

14. absence of the opening into the esophagus

15. inflammation of abdominal serosa

16. downward displacement/prolapse of the entire rectum

17. uncontrolled contractions of the stomach

18. vomiting blood

Activity 8

Word Synthesis/Word Building (continued)

19. incision for removal of stones from the common bile duct

20. resembling tonsils

21. a weakness of the entire stomach

22. pertaining to having pus inside the gallbladder

23. excessive discharge/flow of bile

Activity 8

Word Synthesis/Word Building (continued)

24. surgical removal of the gallbladder

25. hoarseness (difficulty making the sounds of speech)

26. rupture of internal organs

27. without an appetite

28. inflammation around the ileum

Activity 8

Word Synthesis/Word Building (continued)

29. slow digestion

30. difficulty in finding or using the correct words (communicating)

Solutions to Student Practice Activities – Gastrointestinal System

Activity 5

Word Analysis

Number of Components	Prefix	Combining Form(s) Root Stem(s)		Suffix
1. (2)		pharyng		-itis
2. (2)		gingivo		-rrhaphy
3. (3)	peri-	tonsill		-otomy
4. (2)		tonsill		-ectomy
5. (2)		stomato		-plasty
6. (2)		esophag		-ectasis
7. (2)		esophago		-spasm
8. (2)		esophago		-rrhexis
9. (2)		gingiv		-ectomy
10. (2)		pharyng		-algia
11. (2)		pharyngo		-plasty
12. (2)		enter		-ostomy
13. (2)		entero		-rrhexis
14. (2)		duodeno		-cele
15. (3)		entero	colo	-cele
16. (3)	pan-	colo		-megalia
17. (2)		procto		-pexy

Activity 5

Word Analysis (continued)

Number of Components	Prefix	Combining Form(s) Root Stem(s)		Suffix
18. (2)			procto	-scope
19. (2)			sigmoido	-scopy
20. (2)			glosso	-megalia
21. (2)	eu-			-phagia
22. (2)			chole	-lithotomy
23. (2)			cholecysto	-gram
24. (2)			cholangio	-lithiasis
25. (3)		gastro	enter	-ostomy
26. (2)			jejun	-ostomy
27. (2)			chole	-lith (noun suffix)
28. (2)	eu-			-pepsia
29. (2)	an			-osmia
30. (3)	peri-		tonsill	-ar
31. (3)	inter-		dent	-al

Activity 6

Word Analysis for Definition

	Divided Term	Number of Components	Definition
1.	dento/dynia	(2)	toothache
2.	pharyngo/stenosis	(2)	narrowing of throat
3.	pharyng/itis	(2)	inflammation of throat
4.	labio/nasal	(3)	concerning the lips and nose
5.	gingiv/itis	(2)	inflammation of the gums
6.	cheilo/plasty	(2)	reconstruction of oral lips
7.	peri/tonsill/otomy	(3)	incision around the tonsils
8.	tonsill/ectomy	(2)	surgical removal of tonsils
9.	endo/colo/itis	(3)	inflammation of the mucosa of the colon
10.	stomato/plasty	(2)	plastic repair of the mouth
11.	esophag/ectasis	(2)	distention of esophagus
12.	esophago/rrhexis	(2)	rupture of the esophagus
13.	sialo/rrhea	(2)	excessive flow of saliva
14.	sialadeno/edema	(2)	excessive salivary gland tissue fluid
15.	enter/ostomy	(2)	artificial opening of the intestine to the outside through the abdominal wall creating an anus on abdominal wall
16.	colo/enter/ostomy	(3)	anastomosis of the colon and the small intestine
17.	duodeno/cele	(2)	herniation of the duodenum
18.	entero/plegia	(2)	paralysis of some part of the intestines

Activity 6

Word Analysis for Definition (continued)

	Divided Term	Number of Components	Definition
19.	pan/colo/megalia	(3)	enlargement of entire colon
20.	procto/ptosis	(2)	prolapse of the rectum
21.	procto/pexy	(2)	suspension of the rectum
22.	dys/pepsia	(2)	indigestion; painful digestion
23.	dys/osmia	(2)	impaired sense of smell
24.	cholecysto/gram	(2)	x-ray film of gallbladder
25.	intra/dent/al	(3)	concerning within the tooth
26.	gastro/ileo/anastomosis	(3)	surgical joining of the stomach and the ileum
27.	cholecystolith(s)	(2)	stone(s) from the gall bladder
28.	cholecysto/lith(s)	(2)	presence of stone(s) in the gallbladder
29.	cholycysto/lithotomy	(2)	incision into gallbladder for removal of stone(s)
30.	sialadeno/sarcoma	(2)	malignancy of the salivary gland
31.	pharyng/algia	(2)	sore throat
32.	ano/recto/atresia	(3)	absence of opening in rectum and anus
33.	procto/scopy	(2)	examination of rectum/anus with an instrument
34.	pancreato/rrhagia	(2)	blood flow from pancreas
35.	esophago/plegia	(2)	paralysis of esophagus

Activity 7

Combine and Define

Term Formed	Definition
1. subglossitis	infection under the tongue
2. dentodynia	tooth ache
3. intratracheorrhagia	bleeding within the trachea
4. enterospasm	involuntary contractions of the intestines
5. stomatoesophagoplasty	reconstruction of the mouth and esophagus
6. peritonsillitis	inflammation of tissues around the tonsils
7. gingivorrhea	discharge or flow from gingiva
8. dysgastria	painful stomach condition
9. cholecentesis	puncture for aspiration of bile
10. anosmia	inability to sense odors; no sense of smell
11. hypergastrokinesia	excessive movement of stomach
12. anatresia or anoatresia	absence of normal opening of anal orifice
13. panduodenojejunomegalia	the entire duodenum and jejunum are enlarged
14. colostomy	more or less permanent opening of the colon
15. gastrospasm	involuntary contraction of the stomach
16. hemiesophagoplegia	paralysis of one half the esophagus
17. enteroenterostomy	connecting one part of the intestine to another part to form a communication
18. hyposialorrhea	decreased flow of saliva
19. interdental	between the teeth

Activity 7

Combine and Define (continued)

	Term Formed	**Definition**
20.	gastroileoanastomosis	forming a communication between the stomach and ileum
21.	esophagostenosis	narrowing of the esophagus
22.	sialangiectasis	distention of the salivary duct
23.	pharyngodynia	pain in the throat, sore throat
24.	buccocheilolysis	breakdown of the cheeks and lips
25.	hepatectomy	surgical excision of the liver

Activity 8

Word Synthesis/Word Building

1. tooth   ache
   dento   –algia
         dentalgia

2. plastic repair of   mouth   lips
   –plasty   stomato cheilo
        cheilostomatoplasty

3. hemorrhage   pancreas
   –rrhagia, rrhage   pancreato
      pancreatorrhagia, pancreatorrhage

Activity 8

Word Synthesis/Word Building (continued)

4. normal

   eu–

   euphonia

   voice

   –phonia

5. inflammation   within   colon

   –itis   endo–   colo

   endocolitis

6. feces   harden like stones   colon

   feco   –lithiasis   colo

   colofecolithiasis

7. surgical removal   gallbladder

   –ectomy   cholecysto

   cholecystectomy

8. incision into   abdominal wall

   –otomy   laparo

   laparotomy

9. enlargement of   small intestines   large intestines

   –megaly, megalia   entero   colo

   enterocolomegaly, enterocolomegalia

Activity 8

Word Synthesis/Word Building (continued)

10. surgical repair   lip
    –rrhaphy   cheilo
    cheilorrhaphy

11. stones of   salivary gland
    –liths   sialadeno
    sialadenoliths

12. presence of stones   gallbladder
    –lithiasis   cholecysto
    cholecystolithiasis

13. anastomosis of   stomach   duodenum
    –ostomy   gastro   duodeno
    gastroduodenoanastomosis

14. absence of the opening   esophagus
    –atresia   esophagus
    esophagoatresia, esophagatresia

15. inflammation   abdominal serosa
    –itis   peritoneo
    peritonitis

16. downward displacement/prolapse   entire   rectum
    –ptosis   pan–   recto
    panrectoptosis

Activity 8

Word Synthesis/Word Building (continued)

17. uncontrolled contractions of   stomach
    –spasms   gastro
          gastrospasms

18. vomiting   blood
    –emesis   hemo, hemato
          hematemesis

19. incision for removal of stones   common bile duct
    –lithotomy   cholangio
          cholangiolithotomy

20. resembling   tonsils
    –oid   tonsillo
          tonsilloid

21. weakness of the   entire   stomach
    –paresis   pan–   gastro
          pangastroparesis

22. pus   within   gallbladder   concern having
    pyo   intra–   cholecysto   –ic
          intrapyocholecystic

23. excessive   discharge/flow   bile
    hyper–   rrhea   chole
          hypercholerrhea

Activity 8

Word Synthesis/Word Building (continued)

24. excision of/surgical removal   gallbladder
    –ectomy   cholecysto
                cholecystectomy

25. difficulty   sounds of speech
    dys–   –phonia
                dysphonia

26. rupture of   internal organs
    –rrhexis   viscero
                viscerorrhexis

27. without   appetite
    a–, an–   orexia
                anorexia

28. inflammation   around   ileum
    –itis   peri–   ileo
                periileitis

29. slowness (slow)   digestion
    brady–   –pepsia
                bradypepsia

30. difficulty   finding/using words (communicating)
    dys–   –phasia
                dysphasia

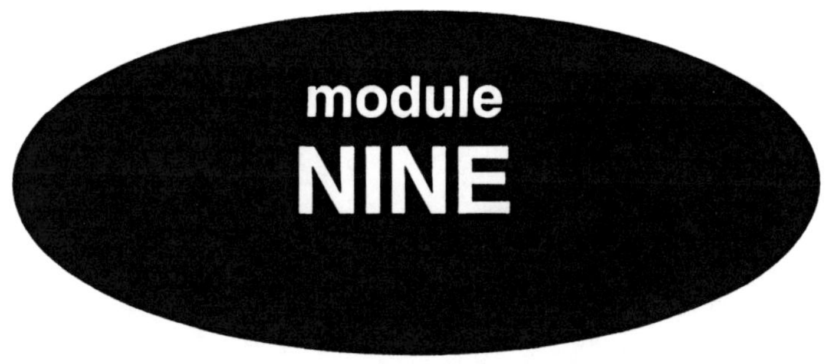

Urinary System

Objectives

Upon completion of these modules the student should be able to:

1. Identify and differentiate prefixes, suffixes, root stems and combining forms of this unit.

2. Write the correctly spelled component, given a list of definitions.

3. Write the definitions for each, given a list of components.

4. Divide the medical term(s) into individual appropriate components; using these definitions, construct a sentence to define the word.

5. Assign the appropriate components to build a medical term when given a medical sentence and construct a correctly spelled medical term.

6. Complete all activities in each module correctly.

The Urinary System

A. Structures and Functions

The structures of the Urinary system are located retroperitoneal and subperitoneal. It consists of two kidneys, two ureters, the urinary bladder and the urethra. The function of this system is to maintain the water balance and acid-base balance of the body, and to form urine and eliminate waste products by excretion of urine. The kidneys filter the blood to remove waste matter and form the urine. The ureters are tubes which convey the urine from the kidneys to the bladder which acts as a reservoir. The urethra is a single tube that conveys the stored urine from the bladder to the outside of the body. In the male this structure is also part of the reproductive system.

B. Components Pertaining to the Urinary System

Combining Form	*Definitions*
1. uro	urinary system, urinary tract, urine
2. nephro	kidney
3. reno	kidney (form rarely used in medical terminology)
4. pyelo	pelvis (renal)
5. uretero	ureter(s)
6. cysto	urinary bladder, a bladder
7. urethro	urethra
8. meato	meatus: an opening or passage

Additional Combining Forms

Combining Form	*Definitions*
9. albumino	albumin
10. calco, calcio	calcium
11. gluco	sugar
12. glyco, glycoso	sugar, sweet
13. litho	stone(s)
14. proteino	protein

Suffixes

15. -cyst	bladder
16. -lith(s)	stone(s)
17. -lithiasis	presence of stones in body
18. -lithotomy	incision for the removal of stone(s)
19. -megalia, -megaly	large, enlarged
20. -tripsy	crushing (intentionally)
21. -uresis	urination: passage of urine voiding
22. -uria	present in urine, urine
23. -ureter(s)	ureter(s): two tubes forming passage for urine from kidneys to bladder
24. -urethra(s)	urethra(s): tube forming passage of urine from bladder to outside

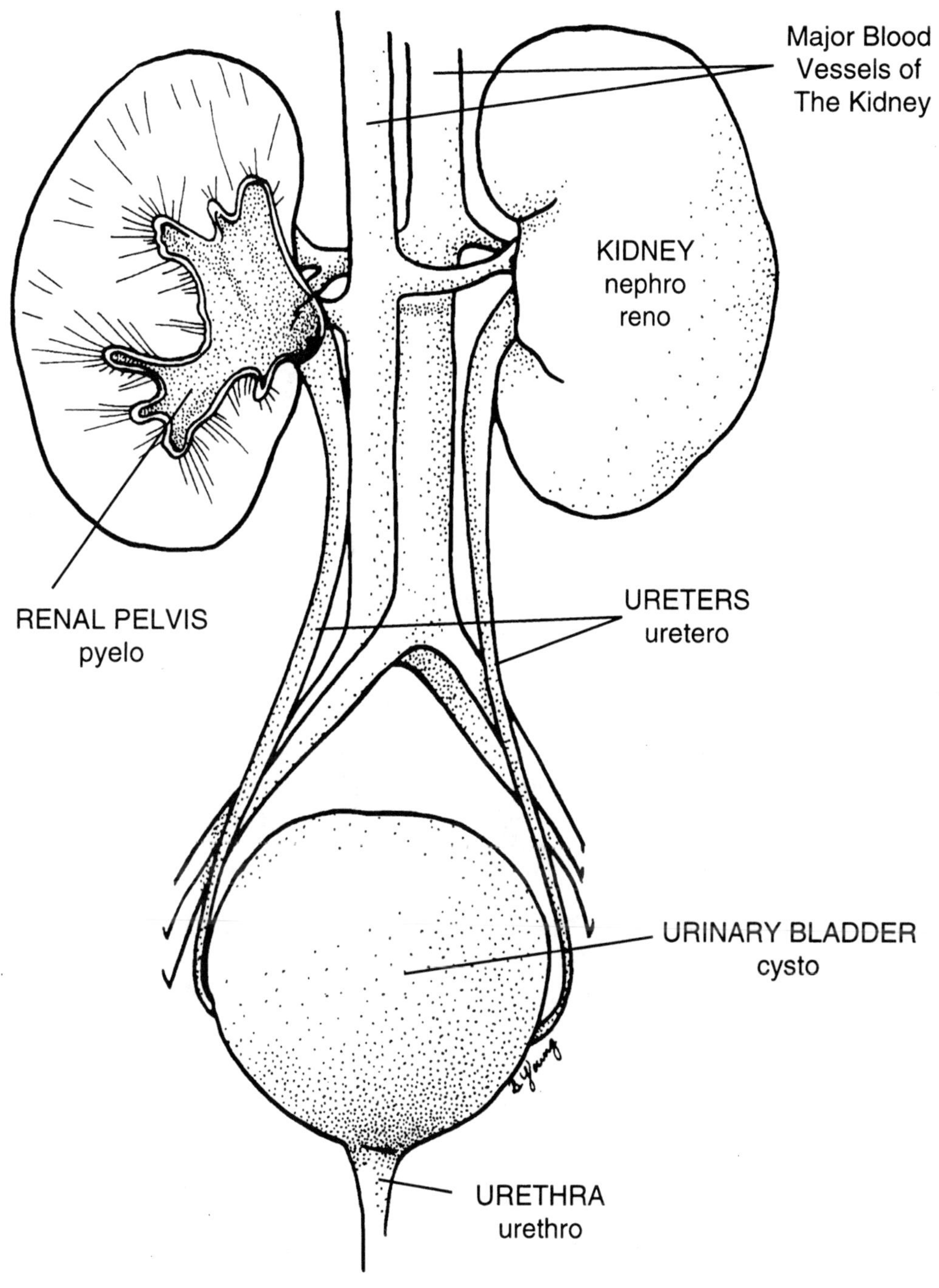

Figure 8.1. Structures of the Urinary System

Student Practice Activities – Urinary System

Activity 1

Flash Cards

Make study cards by printing the new components on one side of the card and definitions on the opposite side. Include all new components from diagram. Check each for correct spelling.

Activity 2

Study Figure 8.1 for new components.

Activity 3

Memorize the new components and their definitions.

Activity 4

Review all suffixes and prefixes of previous modules. Practice reciting/writing definition when reviewing the components. Practice reciting/reviewing components when looking at the definition.

Activity 5

Word Analysis

Divide the following words into components by placing each component in the proper column.

Medical Term	Number of Components	Combining Form(s) Root Stem(s)	Suffix
Example:			
nephrodynia	(2)	nephro	-dynia
1. nephromegalia	( )		
2. nephroptosis	( )		
3. nephrosarcoma	( )		
4. nephropyeloplegia	( )		
5. nephrology	( )		
6. nephrolithiasis	( )		
7. nephroliths	( )		
8. nephroptosia	( )		
9. pyeloplasty	( )		
10. nephrorrhexis	( )		
11. pyelonephrogram	( )		
12. hydroureterosis	( )		
13. pyelonephritis	( )		

Activity 5

Word Analysis (continued)

Medical Term	Number of Components	Combining Form(s) Root Stem(s)	Suffix
14. pyelography	( )		
15. urethrorectal	( )		
16. urethrocystitis	( )		
17. urethrocystotomy	( )		
18. urethrocystostomy	( )		
19. cystectasis	( )		
20. cystomegaly	( )		
21. cystalgia	( )		
22. cystoptosis	( )		
23. cystoparesis	( )		
24. albuminuria	( )		
25. proteinuria	( )		
26. glycosuria	( )		
27. cystoureteroatresia	( )		
28. cystoureterospasm	( )		
29. cystoid	( )		
30. cystoscopy	( )		

Activity 5

Word Analysis (continued)

Divide the following words into Prefix, Combining Form(s) and/or Suffix.

Medical Term	Number of Components	Prefix	Combining Form(s) Root Stems(s)	Suffix
Example:				
dysuria	(2)	dys-		-uria
1. retroperitoneal	( )			
2. pericystic	( )			
3. polycystospasm	( )			
4. anuria	( )			
5. oliguria	( )			
6. transurethral	( )			
7. heminephrectomy	( )			
8. extrarenal	( )			
9. pancystosclerosis	( )			
10. hyperglycosemia	( )			

Activity 6

Combining Components to Form a Word (continued)

Join the components to form properly spelled words.

Prefix	Combining Form(s) Root Stem(s)		Suffix	Correctly Spelled Medical Term
Example:				
	nephro		-algia	nephralgia
1.	nephro		-plasty	__________________________
2.	uretero	pyelo	-cele	__________________________
3.	nephr		-ology	__________________________
4.	nephro		-otomy	__________________________
5.	ureter		-stenosis	__________________________
6.	cysto		-ptosia	__________________________
7.	cyst		-rrhaphy	__________________________
8.	urethro	cysto	-scope	__________________________
9. poly-	cysto		-ic	__________________________
10.	ureter	cyst	-gram	__________________________
11. hemi-	nephro		-ectomy	__________________________
12.	cyst	ureter	-ostomy	__________________________
13.	nephr	uretero	-al	__________________________
14.	cysto	urethro	-genic	__________________________
15. pan-	uro		-plegia	__________________________
16. poly-			-uria	__________________________

Activity 6

Combining Components to Form a Word (continued)

Prefix	Combining Form(s) Root Stem(s)	Suffix	Correctly Spelled Medical Term
17.	proteino	-osis	
18. a-, an-		-uria	
19.	uro	-lith	
20.	albumino	-uria	
21. intra-	cysto	-ic	
22. macro-		-cyst	
23. epi-	cysto	-itis	
24. post-	nephro	-ectomy	
25.	ureter ureter	-ostomy	

Activity 7

Defining Medical Terms

Define these medical terms following the rules for analyzing terms.

Medical Term	Divided Term		Definition
Example:			
nephralgia	nephr (kidney)	-algia (pain)	pain in the kidney, kidney pain
1. nephrotomy			
2. nephropyeloplasty			
3. nephrolithiasis			

Activity 7

Defining Medical Terms (continued)

Medical Term	Divided Term	Definition
4. ureterostenosis		
5. nephrology		
6. ureteropyelocele		
7. cystoptosia		
8. cystopexy		
9. cystorrhaphy		
10. urethrocystoscope		
11. polycystic		
12. ureterocystogram		
13. heminephrectomy		
14. nephroureteral		
15. cystourethrogenic		
16. panuroplegia		
17. polyuria		
18. proteinosis		
19. intracystic		
20. ureteroureterostomy		
21. retroperitoneal		
22. pyocystic		

Activity 7

Defining Medical Terms (continued)

	Medical Term	Divided Term	Definition
23.	cystoid		
24.	hematuria		
25.	uremia		
26.	cystourethroatresia		
27.	polyureterospasms		
28.	glycosuria		
29.	cystorrhexis		
30.	pyelography		
31.	pyelonephrosis		
32.	anuria		
33.	ureterocystoanastomosis		
34.	cystomegaly		
35.	nephrosarcoma		
36.	nephroliths		
37.	nephrolithotomy		
38.	urography		
39.	uroliths		
40.	cystogram		

Activity 8

Word Building from a Sentence

Assign proper components for each idea (definition) within the sentence. Following the rules of combining, write the correct spelling for each medical term formed.

Example:

    sentence: temporary opening of ureter on the abdominal wall
    dividing into definitions:temporary opening   ureter   abdominal wall
    components assigned: -otomy   uretero   laparo
    word formed: ureterolaparotomy

1. kidney pain

2. kidney stones

3. inflammation of the urinary bladder

4. surgical removal of the bladder

Activity 8

Word Building from a Sentence (continued)

5. enlargement of the kidney

6. study of the kidney

7. excision of the kidney

8. rupture of the bladder

9. suture of the ureter

Activity 8

Word Building from a Sentence (continued)

10. cutting of the urethra

11. anastomosis of the bladder and kidney

12. distention of kidney and renal pelvis

13. inflammation of renal pelvis and ureters

14. surgical formation of a communication between the renal pelvis and a ureter

Activity 8

Word Building from a Sentence (continued)

15. instrument used to inspect the bladder

16. paralysis of kidney

17. presence of kidney stones

18. enlarged bladder

19. incision for the removal of stones from the kidneys

Activity 8

Word Building from a Sentence (continued)

20.   dilation of the urethra

21.   prolapsed bladder

22.   suspension of the bladder

23.   painful involuntary contractions of the ureter

24.   pus and blood in the urine

Activity 8

Word Building from a Sentence (continued)

25.   disease of the urinary system

26.   no formation of urine

27.   absence of urination

28.   hardening of the kidney

29.   presence of sugar in the urine

Activity 8

Word Building from a Sentence (continued)

30.   presence of albumin in the urine

Solutions for Practice Activities – Urinary System

Activity 5

Word Analysis

1.	(2)	nephro		-megalia
2.	(2)	nephro		-ptosis
3.	(2)	nephro		-sarcoma
4.	(3)	nephro	pyelo	-plegia
5.	(2)	nephr		-ology
6.	(2)	nephro		-lithiasis
7.	(2)	nephro		-liths
8.	(2)	nephro		-ptosia
9.	(2)	pyelo		-plasty
10.	(2)	nephro		-rrhexis
11.	(3)	pyelo	nephro	-gram
12.	(3)	hydro	ureter	-osis
13.	(3)	pyelo	nephr	-itis
14.	(2)	pyelo		-graphy
15.	(3)	urethro	rect	-al
16.	(3)	urethro	cyst	-itis
17.	(3)	urethro	cyst	-otomy
18.	(3)	urethro	cyst	-ostomy
19.	(2)	cyst		-ectasis

Activity 5

Word Analysis (continued)

20.	(2)	cysto		-megaly
21.	(2)	cyst		-algia
22.	(2)	cysto		-ptosis
23.	(2)	cysto		-paresis
24.	(2)	albumin		-uria
25.	(2)	protein		-uria
26.	(2)	glycos		-uria
27.	(3)	cysto	uretero	-atresia
28.	(3)	cysto	uretero	-spasm
29.	(2)	cyst		-oid
30.	(2)	cysto		-scopy

Divide the words into Prefix, Combining Form(s)/Root Stem, Suffix.

		Prefix	Combining Form(s) Root Stem(s)	Suffix
1.	(3)	retro-	peritone	-al
2.	(3)	peri-	cyst	-ic
3.	(3)	poly-	cysto	-spasm
4.	(2)	an-		-uria
5.	(2)	oligo-		-uria
6.	(3)	trans-	urethr	-al

Activity 5

Word Analysis (continued)

7.	(3)	hemi-	nephr	-ectomy
8.	(3)	extra-	ren	-al
9.	(3)	pan-	cysto	-sclerosis
10.	(3)	hyper-	glycos	-emia

Activity 6

Combining Components to Form a Word

1. nephroplasty
2. ureteropyelocele
3. nephrology
4. nephrotomy
5. ureterostenosis
6. cystoptosia
7. cystorrhaphy
8. urethrocystoscope
9. polycystic
10. ureterocystogram
11. heminephrectomy
12. cystoureterostomy
    cysto-ureterostomy
13. nephroureteral
    nephro-ureteral
14. cystourethrogenic
15. panuroplegia
16. polyuria
17. proteinosis
18. anuria
19. urolith
20. albuminuria
21. intracystic
22. macrocyst
23. epicystitis
24. postnephrectomy
25. ureteroureterostomy
    uretero-ureterostomy

Activity 7

Defining Medical Terms

	Prefix	Combining Form(s) Root Stem(s)		Suffix	Definition
1.		nephr		-otomy	incision into kidney
2.		nephro	pyelo	-plasty	plastic repair of the kidney and renal pelvis
3.		nephro		-lithiasis	presence of stones in kidney
4.		uretero		-stenosis	narrowing of the ureter(s)
5.		nephr		-ology	study of the kidney(s)
6.		uretero	pyelo	-cele	herniation of ureter into renal pelvis
7.		cysto		-ptosia	prolapse of the bladder
8.		cysto		-pexy	suspension of the bladder
9.		cysto		-rrhaphy	suturing of the bladder
10.		urethro	cysto	-scope	instrument used to view urethra and bladder
11.	poly-	cyst		-ic	concerning many fluid filled sacs
12.		uretero	cysto	-gram	x-ray of bladder and ureter(s)
13.	hemi-	nephr		-ectomy	excision of half of a kidney
14.		nephro	ureter	-al	concerning the kidney(s) and ureter(s)
15.		cysto	urethro	-genic	originating in the bladder and urethra
16.	pan-	uro		-plegia	paralysis of entire urinary tract
17.	poly-			-uria	more than normal urine (volume)
18.		protein		-osis	abnormal presence of protein
19.	intra-	cyst		-ic	concerning within the bladder

Activity 7

Defining Medical Terms (continued)

	Combining Form(s) Root Stem(s)		Suffix	Definition
	Prefix			
20.	uretero	ureter	-ostomy	joining of two parts of the ureter for continuous flow of urine
21.	retro-	peritone	-al	pertaining to behind the peritoneum
22.	pyo	cyst	-ic	concerning pus in the bladder
23.	cyst		-oid	resembling a bladder
24.	hemat		-uria	blood in the urine
25.	ur		-emia	urea in the blood (urea: waste product of the body eliminated in the urine)
26.	cysto	urethro	-atresia	absence of a normal opening in the bladder and urethra
27.	poly-	uretero	-spasms	many involuntary ureteral contractions
28.	glycos		-uria	sugar in the urine
29.	cysto		-rrhexis	ruptured bladder
30.	pyelo		-graphy	making an x-ray of the renal pelvis
31.	pyelo	nephr	-osis	disease condition of pelvis of the kidney
32.	an-		-uria	absence of urine
33.	uretero	cysto	-anastomosis	forming a communication between the bladder and ureter
34.	cysto		-megaly	enlarged bladder
35.	nephro		-sarcoma	malignancy of the kidney
36.	nephro		-liths	stones of the kidney

Activity 7

Defining Medical Terms (continued)

	Prefix	Combining Form(s) Root Stem(s)	Suffix	Definition
37.		nephro	-lithotomy	incision to remove kidney stone(s)
38.		uro	-graphy	making an x-ray of the entire or any part of the urinary system
39.		uro	-liths	stones from the urinary system
40.		cysto	-gram	an x-ray picture of the bladder

Activity 8

Word Building from a Sentence

1.	kidney nephro		pain -algia -dynia	nephralgia nephrodynia
2.	kidney nephro		stones -liths	nephroliths
3.	inflammation of -itis		bladder cysto	cystitis
4.	surgical removal of -ectomy		bladder cysto	cystectomy
5.	enlargement of -megalia -megaly		kidney nephro	nephromegalia nephromegaly
6.	study of -ology		kidney nephro	nephrology

Activity 8

Word Building from a Sentence (continued)

7.	excision of	kidney		
	-ectomy	nephro		nephrectomy
8.	rupture of	bladder		
	-rrhexis	cysto		cystorrhexis
9.	suture of	ureter		
	-rrhaphy	uretero		ureterorrhaphy
10.	cutting of	urethra		
	-otomy	urethro		urethrotomy
11.	anastomosis of	bladder	and kidney	
	-anastomosis	cysto	nephro	nephrocystoanastomosis
	-ostomy	cysto	nephro	nephrocystostomy
12.	distention of	kidney	and renal pelvis	
	-extasis	nephro	pyelo	nephropyelectasis
	-extasia			nephropyelectasia
13.	inflammation of	renal pelvis	ureters	
	-itis	pyelo	uretero	pyeloureteritis
14.	surgical formation of a communication	renal pelvis	ureter	
	-anastomosis	pyelo	uretero	pyeloureteroanastomosis
	-ostomy	pyelo	uretero	pyeloureterostomy
15.	instrument used to inspect	urinary bladder		
	-scope	cysto		cystoscope
16.	paralysis of	kidney		
	-plegia	nephro		nephroplegia
17.	presence of stones	kidney		
	-lithiasis	nephro		nephrolithiasis

Activity 8

Word Building from a Sentence (continued)

18.	enlarged -megaly -megalia	bladder cysto		cystomegaly cystomegalia
19.	incision for removal of stones -lithotomy	kidney nephro		nephrolithotomy
20.	dilation of -ectasis -ectasia	urethra urethro		urethrectasis urethrectasia
21.	prolapsed -ptosis -ptosia	bladder cysto		cystoptosis cystoptosia
22.	suspension of -pexy	bladder cysto		cystopexy
23.	painful -dys	involuntary contractions -spasm	ureter uretero	dysureterospasms
24.	blood hemato	in the urine -uria	pus pyo	pyohematuria hemopyuria
25.	disease of -pathy	urinary system uro		uropathy
26.	no formation of a-, an-	urine -uria		anuria
27.	absence of a-, an-	urination -uresis		anuresis
28.	hardening of -sclerosis	kidney nephro		nephrosclerosis

Activity 8

Word Building from a Sentence (continued)

29. present in urine   sugar
    -uria   glyco, glycoso   glycosuria

30. present in urine   albumin
    -uria   albumino   albuminuria

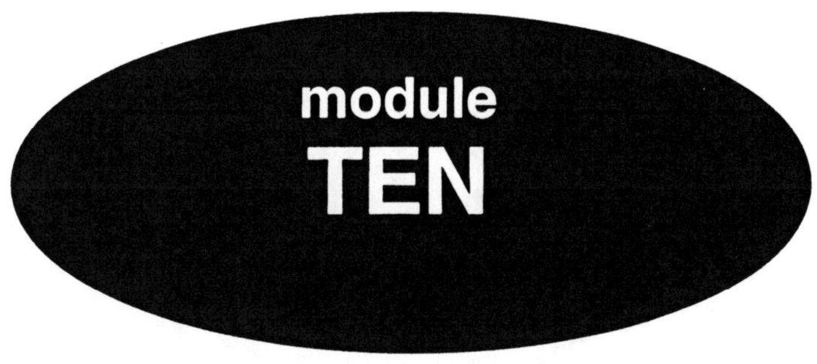

Male Reproductive System

Objectives

Upon completion of these modules the student should be able to:

1. Identify and differentiate prefixes, suffixes, root stems and combining forms of this unit.

2. Write the correctly spelled component, given a list of definitions.

3. Write the definitions for each, given a list of components.

4. Divide the medical term(s) into individual appropriate components; using these definitions, construct a sentence to define the word.

5. Assign the appropriate components to build a medical term when given a medical sentence and construct a correctly spelled medical term.

6. Complete all activities in each module correctly.

The Male Reproductive System

A. Structures and Functions

The male reproductive system is primarily for procreation (the act of creating new life), but some structures also function with other systems. The two testes produce spermatozoa for procreation and as an endocrine gland for the production of male sex hormone – testosterone. The testes are enclosed in a sac called the scrotum. Tubular structures transport the spermatozoa from the testes to the urethra with fluids secreted by the glands and ducts along the way. These tubules include the epididymis (responsible for spermatogenesis), vas deferens, seminal duct, ejaculatory duct and the urethra. The urethra functions to convey from the body not only the urine but also the semen, which is the fluid of the glands and ducts containing the spermatozoa. The prostate gland is an accessory organ which also contributes fluid to the semen. The penis is a hollow tubular structure. The urethra forms the central canal to convey urine and semen to the outside. The penis is the male organ of copulation (sexual intercourse). Gonads refer to both the male or female sex glands. Genitals (genitalia) refer to the reproductive organs, especially the external organs, of both the male and female.

B. Components Pertaining to the Male Reproductive System

Combining Form	Definition
1. andro	man, male
viri	male, masculine
	represented by the symbol ♂
2. peno	penis
phallo	
3. balano	glans penis
4. prepuco	prepuce: foreskin

Combining Form	*Definition*
5. vaso	inclusive component for sperm carrying internal tubular structures. In the male: vas deferens, seminal ducts, ejaculatory ducts
6. prostato	prostate gland
7. orchio orchido testo	testis, sing. (testes, pl.)
testiculo	testicle(s)
8. epididymo	epididymis
9. scroto	scrotum
10. genito genitalia	reproductive organs
11. spermatazoo	spermatozoa, pl., spermatozoon, sing. mature male sex cell formed within the testes

Additional Components

Prefixes

12. circum- *	around, on all sides
13. crypto- **	hidden, a recessed chamber

Suffixes

14. -cision	to cut, cutting
15. -ligation	procedure for tying
16. -ism	state of, condition of

* Circumcision literally means "to cut around". This term is commonly accepted as "the removal of the prepuce" but may refer to the rare practice of female circumcision, the partial or complete removal of the clitoris.

** Does not follow the usual rule of prefixes. When combining with components beginning with "o", crypto drops the "o" ending.

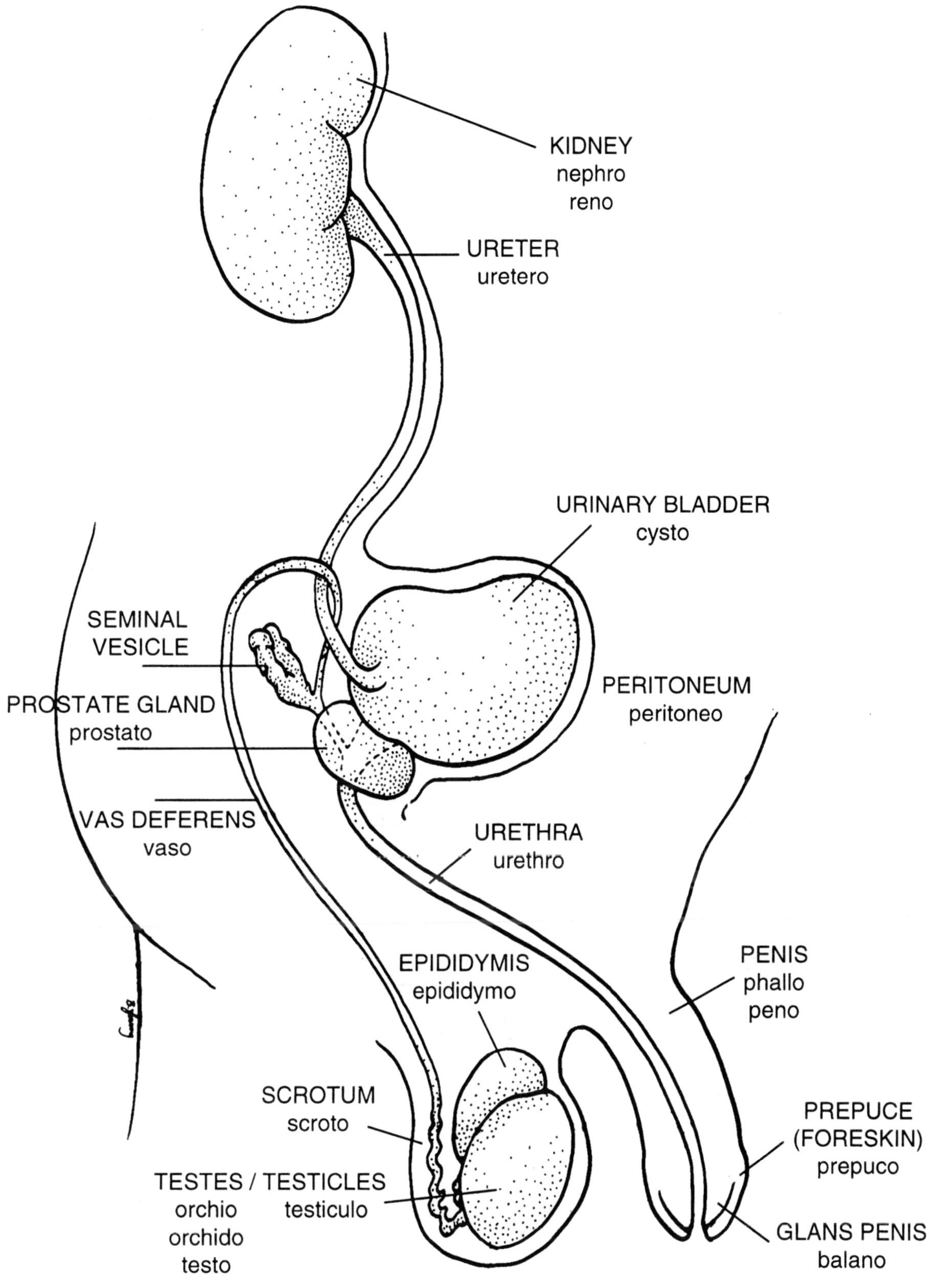

Figure 9.1. Lateral View of the Male Genitourinary System

Student Practice Activities – Male Reproductive System

Activity 1

Flash Cards

Make flash cards, a separate card for each component, as in previous modules. Make sure each is correctly spelled.

Activity 2

Study Figure 9.1 for new components.

Activity 3

Memorize new components and their definitions.

Activity 4

Review all suffixes and prefixes of previous modules. Practice reciting/writing definitions when reviewing components. Practice reciting/writing correct component spelling.

Activity 5

Word Analysis

Divide the following words into components by placing components in the proper column.

Medical Term	Number of Components	Prefix	Combining Form(s) Root Stems(s)	Suffix
Example: panorchiectomy	(3)	pan-	orchi	-ectomy
1. balanalgia	( )			
2. balanomegalia	( )			
3. balanolysis	( )			
4. balanorrhage	( )			
5. balanotomy	( )			
6. hemiorchidectomy	( )			
7. panpenectomy	( )			
8. orchiodynia	( )			
9. orchiotomy	( )			
10. orchiopexy	( )			
11. anorchism	( )			
12. scrotocele	( )			
13. androids	( )			
14. pyoprostatorrhea	( )			
15. testiculosclerosis	( )			

Activity 5

Word Analysis (continued)

Medical Term	Number of Components	Prefix	Combining Form(s) Root Stems(s)	Suffix
16. vasoligation	( )			
17. phallomegalia	( )			
18. prepucostenosis	( )			
19. urethratresia	( )			
20. penorrhexis	( )			
21. vasorrhaphy	( )			
22. vasoepididymostomy	( )			
23. cryptorchism	( )			
24. vasoepididymoanastomosis	( )			
25. polyorchidism	( )			
26. unilateral orchiectomy	( )			
27. anorchidism	( )			
28. prostatomegalia	( )			
29. prostatocystitis	( )			
30. prostatolithiasis	( )			

Activity 6

Word Building From a Sentence

Join the components to form properly spelled words.

Prefix	Combining Form(s) Root Stem(s)	Suffix	Correctly Spelled Medical Term
Example:			
	balano	-rrhea	balanorrhea
1.	balano	-rrhagia	
2.	prepuco urethro	-stenosis	
3.	prostato cysto	-cele	
4.	testiculo	-lysis	
5. pan-	genito	-plasty	
6.	vaso orchio	-rrhaphy	
7. dys-		-uria	
8. a-, an-	spermato	-poiesis	
9.	scroto	-sclerosis	
10. peri-	orchido	-itis	
11.	prepuco	-ectomy	
12.	vaso -anastomosis		
13.	vaso vaso	-ostomy	
14. a-, an-	orchio	-ism	
15. poly-	orchido	-ism	
16.	andro	-genic	

Activity 6

Word Building From a Sentence (continued)

	Prefix	Combining Form(s) Root Stem(s)	Suffix	Correctly Spelled Medical Term
17.		vaso	-ligation	
18.	bi-, latero-		-al	
		orchio	-ectomy	
19.		urethro	-lithiasis	
20.		hemo	-urethra	
21.		balano	-megalia	
22.		prepuco	-lysis	
23.		prostato	-itis	
24.	trans-	vaso	-otomy	
25.		scroto	-centesis	
26.		genito	-dynia	
27.		prostato	-sarcoma	
28.		orchido	-oma	
29.		vaso	-plegia	
30.		phallo	-rrhexis	

Activity 7

Defining Medical Terms

Define these medical terms following the rules for analyzing terms.

Medical Term	Divided Term	Definition
Example: balanorrhea	balano -rrhea	a flow from the glans penis
1. balanopyorrhagia		
2. phallorrhexis		
3. prostatocystocele		
4. testiculolysis		
5. pangenitoplasty		
6. vaso-orchiorrhaphy / vasoorchiorrhaphy		
7. dysuria		
8. aspermatopoiesis		
9. scrotosclerosis		
10. periorchitis / periorchiitis		
11. prepucectomy		
12. vasoanastomosis		
13. vasovasostomy		
14. anorchism		
15. polyorchidism		

Activity 7

Defining Medical Terms (continued)

Medical Term	Divided Term	Definition
16. android		
17. vasoligation		
18. bilateral orchiectomy		
19. urethrolithiasis		
20. balanoplasty		
21. balanomegalia		
22. prepucolysis		
23. prostatitis		
24. transvasotomy		
25. scrotocentesis		
26. genitodynia		
27. prostatosarcoma		
28. orchidoma		
29. vasoplegia		
30. prepucourethrostenosis		

Activity 8

Word Building From a Sentence

Assign proper components for each idea (definition) within the sentence. Following the rules of combining, write the correct spelling of each medical term formed.

Example:

sentence:	inflammation of	the prepuce
dividing into definitions:	inflammation of	prepuce
components assigned:	-itis	prepuco
word formed:	prepucitis	

1. reconstruction of the genitalia

2. bloody flow from the urethra

3. inflammation of the glans penis

Activity 8

Word Building From a Sentence (continued)

4. rupture of the scrotum

5. enlargement of the penis

6. incision of the vas deferens

7. absence of testes

8. condition of having more than two testes

Activity 8

Word Building From a Sentence (continued)

9. hidden testes

10. anastomosis of two parts of the vas deferens

11. surgical removal of the prostate and bladder

12. suspension of the testes

13. narrowing of the urethra

Activity 8

Word Building From a Sentence (continued)

14.   absence of an opening between the vas deferens and the urethra

15.   the tying of the vas deferens for sterilization

16.   the cutting out of all or part of the vas deferens

17.   puncture for aspiration of fluid from the scrotum

18.   surgical excision of both testes

Activity 8

Word Building From a Sentence (continued)

19. freeing up of the ejaculatory duct

20. pus and blood in the urethra

21. inflammation of the testes and epididymis

22. herniation of the scrotum

23. resembling man

Activity 8

Word Building From a Sentence (continued)

24. disease of the testes

25. presence of stones in the prostate

26. incision into prostate gland for removal of stones

27. prostate stones (not in the body)

28. pain in the penis

Activity 8

Word Building From a Sentence (continued)

29. absence of genitalia

30. undescended testicles

Solutions for Practice Activities – Male Reproductive System

Activity 5

Word Analysis

	Number of Components	Prefix	Combining Form(s) Root Stem(s)	Suffix
1.	(2)		balan	-algia
2.	(2)		balano	-megalia
3.	(2)		balano	-lysis
4.	(2)		balano	-rrhage
5.	(2)		balan	-otomy
6.	(3)	hemi-	orchid	-ectomy
7.	(3)	pan-	pen	-ectomy
8.	(2)		orchio	-dynia
9.	(2)		orchi	-otomy
10.	(2)		orchio	-pexy
11.	(3)	an-	orchi	-ism
12.	(2)		scroto	-cele
13.	(2)		andr	-oids
14.	(3)		pyo prostato	-rrhea
15.	(2)		testiculo	-sclerosis
16.	(2)		vaso	-ligation
17.	(2)		phallo	-megalia

Activity 5

Word Analysis (continued)

Number of Components	Prefix	Combining Form(s) Root Stem(s)		Suffix
18. (2)		prepuco		-stenosis
19. (2)		urethr		-atresia
20. (2)		peno		-rrhexis
21. (2)		vaso		-rrhaphy
22. (3)		vaso	epididym	-ostomy
23. (3)	crypt-	orchi		-ism
24. (3)		vaso	epididymo	-anastomosis
25. (3)	poly-	orchid		-ism
26. (3)	uni-	later		-al
(2)		orchi		-ectomy
27. (3)	an-	orchido		-ism
28. (2)		prostato		-megalia
29. (3)		prostato	cyst	-itis
30. (2)		prostato		-lithiasis

Activity 6

Word Building

1. balanorrhagia
2. prepucourethrostenosis
   prepuco-urethrostenosis
3. prostatocystocele
4. testiculolysis
5. pangenitoplasty
6. vasoorchiorrhaphy
   vaso-orchiorrhaphy
7. dysuria
8. aspermatopoiesis
9. scrotosclerosis
10. periorchiditis
11. prepucectomy
12. vasoanastomosis
13. vasovasostomy
14. anorchism
15. polyorchidism
    polyorchism
16. androgenic
17. vasoligation
18. bilateral orchiectomy
19. urethrolithiasis
20. hemourethra
21. balanomegalia
22. prepucolysis
23. prostatitis
24. transvasotomy
25. scrotocentesis
26. genitodynia
27. prostatosarcoma
28. orchidoma
29. vasoplegia
30. phallorrhexis

Activity 7

Defining Medical Terms

1.	balano	pyo	-rrhegia	discharge of pus and bloody flow from glans penis
2.	phallo		-rrhexis	ruptured penis
3.	prostato	cysto	-cele	herniation of prostate into bladder
4.	testiculo		-lysis	freeing up of testes; breakdown of testes
5.	pan-	genito	-plasty	plastic repair of all the genitalia
6.	vaso	orchio	-rrhaphy	suturing of vas deferens and testes
7.	dys-		-uria	painful urination; difficulty urinating
8.	a-	spermato	-poiesis	no production of sperm
9.	scroto		-sclerosis	hardening of the scrotum
10.	peri-	orchi	-itis	inflammation around the testes
11.	prepuc		-ectomy	excision of prepuce; circumcision
12.		vaso	-anastomosis	joining two parts of the vas deferens
13.	vaso	vas	-ostomy	anastomosis of two parts of vas deferens
14.	an-	orchi	-ism	condition of having no testes, (acquired or congenital)
15.	poly-	orchid	-ism	having more than two testes
16.	andr		-oid	resembling man
17.	vaso		-ligation	tying of the vas deferens
18.	bi-	latero orchi	-al -ectomy	surgical removal of both testes (from both sides)
19.	urethro		-lithiasis	stone(s) in the urethra
20.	balano		-plasty	reconstruction of glans penis, plastic repair of glans penis

Activity 7

Defining Medical Terms (continued)

21.	balano		-megalia	large glans penis
22.	prepuco		-lysis	freeing up or break down of prepuce
23.	prostat		-itis	inflammation of prostate gland
24.	trans-	vas	-otomy	cutting across the vas deferens
25.	scroto		-centesis	tapping of the scrotum
26.	genito		-dynia	pain in the genitalia
27.	prostato		-sarcoma	cancer of the prostate gland
28.	orchid		-oma	tumor of the testes
29.	vaso		-plegia	paralysis of the vas deferens
30.	prepuco	urethro	-stenosis	narrowing of the prepuce and urethra

Activity 8

Word Building From a Sentence

1.	reconstruction of -plasty	genitalia genito	genitoplasty
2.	bloody flow -rrhage -rrhagia	urethra urethro	urethrorrhage urethrorrhagia
3.	inflammation of -itis	glans penis balano	balanitis
4.	rupture of -rrhexis	scrotum scroto	scrotorrhexis

Activity 8

Word Building From a Sentence (continued)

5.	enlargement of -megalia -megaly	penis phallo or peno		phallomegalia; penomegalia
6.	incision of -otomy	vas deferens vaso		vasotomy
7.	absence of a-, an-	testes orchio or orchido		anorchism; anorchidism
8.	condition of having -ism	more than two (normal number) poly-	testes orchio or orchido	polyorchism; polyorchidism
9.	hidden crypto-	testes orchio orchido	(state of having) -ism	cryptorchism cryptorchidism
10.	anastomosis of -anastomosis	vas deferens vaso		vasoanastomosis
11.	surgical removal -ectomy	prostate prostato	bladder cysto	prostatocystectomy
12.	suspension of -pexy	testes orchio orchido testo		orchiopexy orchidopexy testopexy
13.	narrowing of -stenosis	urethra urethro		urethrostenosis
14.	absence of opening -atresia	vas deferens vaso	urethra urethro	urethrovasoatresia; urethrovasatresia vaso-urethroatresia

Activity 8

Word Building From a Sentence (continued)

15.	tying of -ligation	vas deferens vaso		vasoligation
16.	cutting out (surgical removal of) -ectomy	vas deferens vaso		vasectomy
17.	puncture for aspiration -centesis	fluid hydro	scrotum scroto	hydroscrotocentesis
18.	surgical excision -ectomy	both pan-	testes testo orchio orchido	pantestectomy panorchiectomy panorchidectomy
19.	freeing up -lysis	vas deference vaso		vasolysis
20.	pus pyo	blood hemo hemato	urethra urethro	hematopyourethra hemopyourethra
21.	inflammation of -itis	testes orchio orchido testo	epididymis epididymo	orchioepididymitis orchio-epididymitis testoepididymitis testo-epididymitis
22.	herniation of -cele	scrotum scroto		scrotocele
23.	resembling -oid	man andro		android

Activity 8

Word Building From a Sentence (continued)

24.	disease of	testes		
	-pathy	orchido		orchidopathy
		orchio		orchiopathy
		testo		testopathy
25.	presence of stones	prostate		
	-lithiasis	prostato		prostatolithiasis
26.	incision to remove stones	prostate gland		
	-lithotomy	prostato		prostatolithotomy
27.	prostate	stones		
	prostato	-liths		prostatoliths
28.	pain	penis		
	-algia	peno		penalgia
	-dynia	phallo		penodynia
				phallalgia
				phallodynia
29.	absence of	genitalia		
	a-, an-	-genitalia		agenitalia
30.	undescended	testicles	(state of)	
	crypto-	orchio	-ism	cryptorchism
		orchido		cryptorchidism

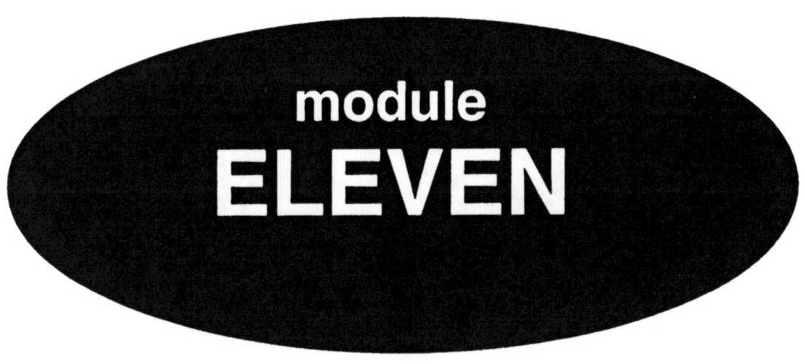

Female Reproductive System

Objectives

Upon completion of these modules the student should be able to:

1. Identify and differentiate prefixes, suffixes, root stems and combining forms of this unit.

2. Write the correctly spelled component, given a list of definitions.

3. Write the definitions for each, given a list of components.

4. Divide the medical term(s) into individual appropriate components; using these definitions, construct a sentence to define the word.

5. Assign the appropriate components to build a medical term when given a medical sentence and construct a correctly spelled medical term.

6. Complete all activities in each module correctly.

The Female Reproductive System

A. Structures and Functions

The organs of the female reproductive system function primarily for reproduction, but as in the male reproductive system, the glands function to effect other systems of the body.

The two ovaries produce ova (the female eggs sex cells). As the testes are the gonads of the male, the ovaries are the female gonads and serve both the reproductive and the endocrine systems. Estrogen and progesterone are two hormones produced by ovaries.

The uterine tubes convey the ova from the ovaries to the uterus. It is in these tubes that fertilization of the ova usually occurs. The uterus is the organ of containment for the product of conception (the fertilized ovum). The fertilized ovum attaches to and grows within the uterus. This period of growth and development of this product of conception, called pregnancy. The non-pregnant uterus prepares each month for this event. When no fertilized ovum is present the uterus sheds its lining to start the process again. This process of shedding is called menstruation.

All of the above are internal structures. They may not be viewed from the outside without instrumentation.

The cervix is the external neck portion of the uterus.

The vagina is considered external since it may be seen and examined without instruments. This tubular structure is the receptor of the penis during copulation and forms the birth canal a passageway for the fetus, from the uterus to the outside.

The vulva are the external lips of the genitalia.

B. Components Pertaining to the Female Reproductive System

Combining Forms	*Definition*
1. gyneco gyne gyno	woman, women symbol for woman ♀
2. pelvi pelvo	pelvic cavity containing the reproductive organs
3. oophoro ovario	ovary (ovaries, pl.)
4. oo	ovum (ova, pl.), egg(s)
5. salpingo	salpinx (salpinges, pl.): also called uterine tubes, fallopian tubes, oviducts
6. hystero	uterus
7. utero	uterus, usually use as an anatomical reference
8. metro, metrio -metrium (noun suffix)	uterus, usually refers to the muscle uterine structure
9. perimetrio	perimetrium: serosa of the uterus, tissue which covers the outside of the uterus
10. myometrio	myometrium: muscle of the uterus
11. endometrio	endometrium: mucosal lining lining of the uterus, mucosa of the uterus
12. cervico trachelo	uterine cervix, the neck of the uterus. Both components may refer to the neck either that connecting the head and the trunk or to the uterine cervix.
13. colpo vagino	vagina
14. vulvo	vulva; in anatomy: labia majora
15. perineo	perineum: the tissue forming the floor of the pelvic cavity located between the vulva and the rectum in the female. In the male it is the area between the rectum and the scrotum.
16. episio	term indicating the perineum and/or the vulva
17. meno	menstruation, menses (literally, monthly)

C. Components Pertaining to Pregnancy and Birth

Combining Forms	*Definition*
18. atelo	incomplete
19. amnio	amniotic fluid, fluid in pregnant uterus surrounding the fetus
20. feto	the fetus
21. -gravid	pregnant, pregnancy (gravid)
22. -gravida	pregnant woman (gravida)
23. multi-	many, much
24. -natal	pertaining to birth, birthday -nate (natal)
25. neo-	new, recent
26. nulli-	never, none
27. -para	woman having carried a viable (para) (living) fetus beyond the 20th week of pregnancy regardless of whether it was alive at birth
28. pedo pedio	child, children
29. primi-	first, one
30. toco, toko	birth, process of birth
31. -tocia	process of birth, labor

D. Vocabulary

1. embryo	products of conception from 2 to 8 weeks in utero; usually too immature to sustain life outside the uterus.
2. fetus	product of conception from 8+ weeks to birth, still in utero
3. pelvis	a basin-like structure; may refer to the renal or the reproductive pelvis
4. viable	capable of living outsides the uterus

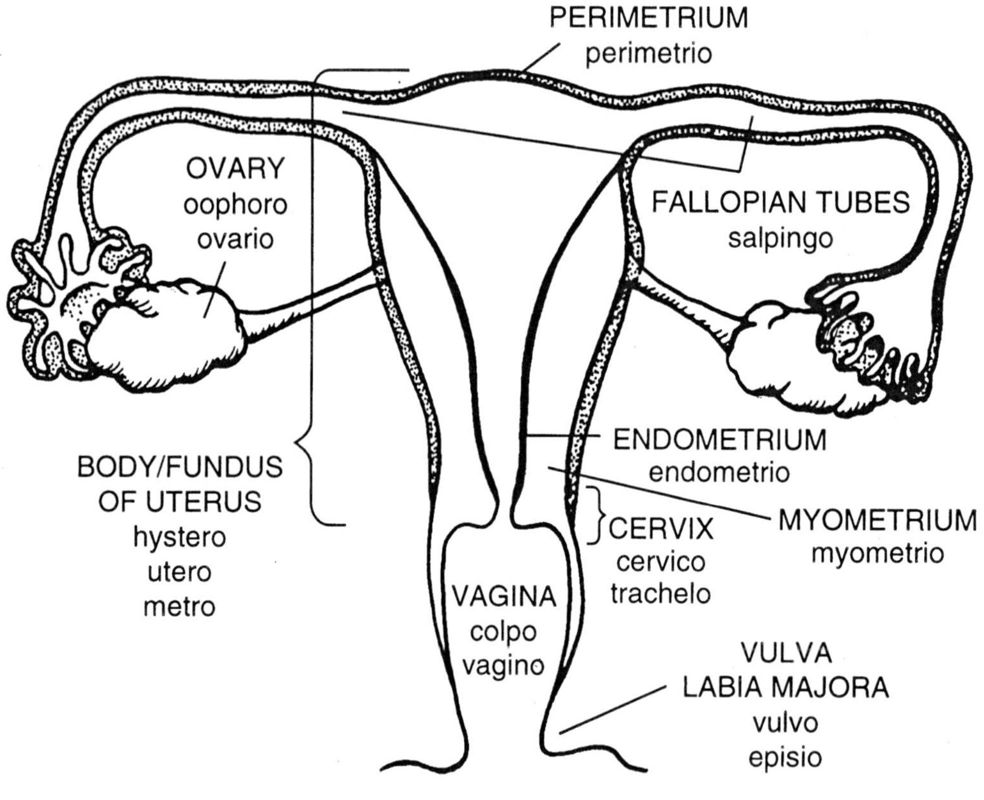

Figure 10.1. Internal Female Reproductive Organs

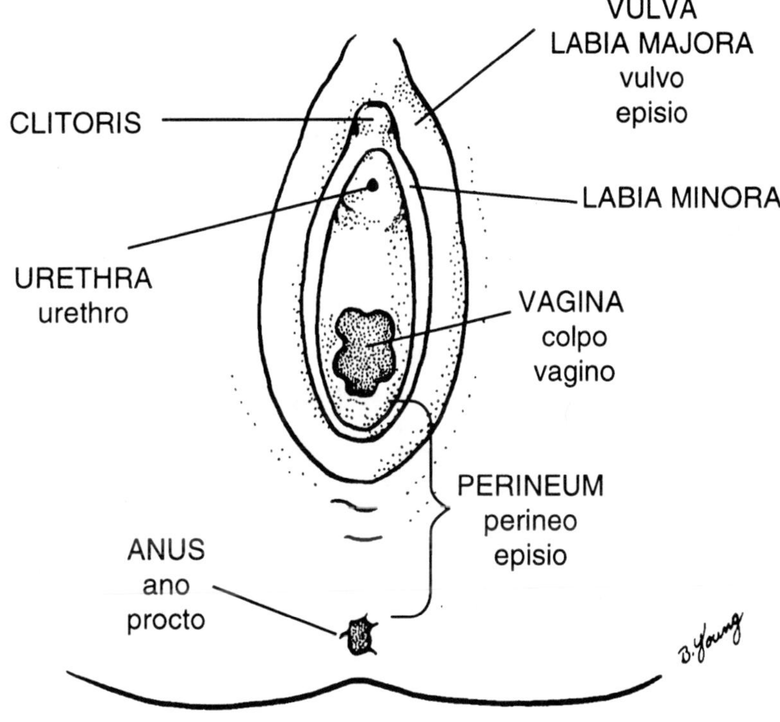

Figure 10.2. Perineal View of Female External Genitalia

Student Activities – Female Reproductive System

Activity 1

Flash Cards

Make flash cards, a separate card for each component, as in the previous modules. Make sure each is correctly spelled.

Activity 2

Study Figures (10.1-2) for new component.

Activity 3

Memorize new components and vocabulary and their definitions.

Activity 4

Review all suffixes and prefixes of previous modules. Practice reciting/writing component definitions. Practice reciting/writing correct component spelling. Review vocabulary.

Student Practice Activities

Activity 5

Word Analysis

Divide the following words into components by placing components in the proper column.

Medical Term	Number of Components	Prefix	Combining Form(s) Root Stems(s)	Suffix
Example: colpotomy	(2)		colpo	-otomy
1. oophorocentesis	( )			
2. ovariocentesis	( )			
3. salpingitis	( )			
4. salpingorrhexis	( )			
5. salpingouterostomy	( )			
6. salpingectomy	( )			
7. salpingoptosis	( )			
8. salpingo-oophoropexy	( )			
9. salpingo-oophoroplasty	( )			
10. colpopexy	( )			
11. colporrhaphy	( )			
12. colposcope	( )			
13. vaginitis	( )			

Activity 5

Word Analysis (continued)

Medical Term	Number of Components	Prefix	Combining Form(s) Root Stems(s)	Suffix
14. cervicocolpoplasty	( )			
15. trachelitis	( )			
16. trachelodynia	( )			
17. cervicalgia	( )			
18. panhysterectomy	( )			
19. salpingo-oophorectomy	( )			
20. menorrhea	( )			
21. panoophorosalpingohysterectomy	( )			
22. intravaginal	( )			
23. endovaginal	( )			
24. amenorrhea	( )			
25. oocyst	( )			
26. oogenic	( )			
27. dystocia	( )			
28. multipara	( )			
29. primipara	( )			
30. perimetriectomy	( )			
31. pyosalpinx	( )			

Activity 5

Word Analysis (continued)

Medical Term	Number of Components	Prefix	Combining Form(s) Root Stems(s)	Suffix
32. vaginohysterotokotomy	( )			
33. atocia	( )			
34. colposarcoma	( )			
35. dysmenorrhea	( )			

Activity 6

Word Building

Join the components to form a properly spelled word.

Components			Correctly Spelled Medical Term
Example:			
vagino	vulvo	-rrhaphy	vaginovulvorrhaphy
1. hyster	cervico	-ectomy	
2. colpo	cervico	-ostomy	
3. hyster	-rrhexis		
4. oligo-	meno	-rrhea	
5. oo	oophor	-centesis	
6. dys-	men	-rrhea	
7. hystero	salping	-pexy	

Activity 6

Word Building (continued)

Join the components to form a properly spelled word.

Components				Correctly Spelled Medical Term
8.	hyster	salping	-ptosis	
9.	hemo	salpingo		
10.	salpingo	hyster	-anastomosis	
11.	trachel	myometrio	-rrhaphy	
12.	pan-	hystero	-ectomy	
13.	oo	oophoro	-otomy	
14.	endometrio		-lysis	
15.	trachelo		-atresia	
16.	myometrio	-oma		
17.	cervico	-sarcoma		
18.	endo-	cervico	-itis	
19.	intra-	trachelo	therapy	
20.		embryo	-ology	
21.	intra-	utero	pyo	-osis
22.	colpo	cervico	-dynia	
23.	lapar	hyster	toco	-otomy
24.	genito	path	-ology	
25.	colpo	vulvo	cervico	-plasty

Activity 7

Defining Medical Terms

Define these medical terms following the rules for analyzing terms.

Medical Term	Divided Term	Definition
Example: colporrhaphy	colpo -rrhapy	suturing of the vagina
1. colpopexy		
2. colpoptosis		
3. salpingo-oophoroplasty		
4. salpingorrhagia		
5. salpingorrhexis		
6. salpingo-uterostomy		
7. salpingo-oophoropexy		
8. ovariocentesis		
9. oophorocentesis		
10. colposcope		
11. salpingitis		
12. vaginitis		
13. salpingoptosis		
14. cervicocolpoplasty		
15. salpingectomy		
16. gynecology		

Activity 7

Defining Medical Terms (continued)

Medical Term	Divided Term	Definition
17. cervicalgia		
18. proctocolpocele		
19. amenorrhea		
20. trachelitis		
21. endovaginal		
22. panhysterectomy		
23. intravaginal		
24. salpingo-oophorectomy		
25. panoophorosalpingohysterectomy		
26. endometriolysis		
27. perineotomy		
28. menorrhea		
29. episiotomy		
30. dysmenorrhea		
31. ookinesis		
32. atocia		
33. dystocia		
34. neonatal		
35. vaginohysterotokotomy		

Activity 7

Defining Medical Terms (continued)

Medical Term	Divided Term	Definition
36. multipara		
37. hemimyometrioplegia		
38. nulligravida		
39. pyosalpinx		
40. perimetriectomy		
41. colpostenosis		
42. oogenic		
43. primipara		
44. trachelodynia		
45. uteroparesis		

Activity 8

Word Building from a Sentence

Assign proper components for each idea (definition) within the sentence. Following the rules of combining, write the correct spelling of each medical term.

Example:

sentence: surgical excision of the ovaries

divide into definitions: surgical excision ovaries – there are only two ovaries, component needed for "all"

components: -ectomy oophoro pan-

word formed: panoophorectomy

1. excision of the entire uterus (including the cervix)

2. formation of a communication between the vagina and cervix

3. rupture of the uterus

Activity 8

Word Building from a Sentence(continued)

4. scanty menstrual flow

5. breakdown of the endometrium

6. incision into the ovary for an egg

7. blood in both fallopian tubes

8. joining the uterus with the salpinges – only two oviducts, hence component for all needed

Activity 8

Word Building from a Sentence(continued)

9. sewing the cervix and the muscle of the uterus

10. a prolapse or downward displacement of the uterus

11. puncture of the ovary for aspiration of an ovum

12. painful menstrual flow, "cramps"

13. suspension of the uterus and fallopian tubes

Activity 8

Word Building from a Sentence (continued)

14.　suturing of the vagina and labia majora

15.　rupture of the inside (lining) of the oviduct

16.　reconstruction of the vagina, vulva and the cervix

17.　herniation of the bladder into the vagina

18.　cervical cancer, malignant tumor of the cervix

Activity 8

Word Building from a Sentence (continued)

19. tumor of the uterine muscle

20. inflammation within the cervix (lining)

21. abnormal condition of having pus inside the uterus

22. pain in the vagina and cervix

23. cutting through the abdominal wall and uterus to deliver a child

Activity 8

Word Building from a Sentence (continued)

24. excision of the entire uterus and cervix

____

____

____

25. absence of a normal opening into the cervix

____

____

Solutions to Practice Activities – Female Reproductive System

Activity 5

Word Analysis

Number of Components	Prefix	Combining Form(s) Root Stem(s)		Suffix
1. (2)		oophoro		-centesis
2. (2)		ovario		-centesis
3. (2)		salping		-itis
4. (2)		salpingo		-rrhexis
5. (3)	salpingo		uter	-ostomy
6. (2)		salping		-ectomy
7. (2)		salpingo		-ptosis
8. (3)	salpingo		oophoro	-pexy
9. (3)	salpingo		oophoro	-plasty
10. (2)		colpo		-pexy
11. (2)		colpo		-rrhaphy
12. (2)		colpo		-scope
13. (2)		vagin		-itis
14. (3)	cervico		colpo	-plasty
15. (2)		trachel		-itis
16. (2)		trachel		-dynia
17. (2)		cervic		-algia

Activity 5

Word Analysis (continued)

Number of Components	Prefix	Combining Form(s) Root Stem(s)			Suffix
18. (3)	pan-	hyster			-ectomy
19. (3)		salpingo		oophor	-ectomy
20. (2)		meno			-rrhea
21. (5)	pan-	oophoro	salpingo	hyster	-ectomy
22. (3)	intra-	vagin			-al
23. (3)	endo-	vagin			-al
24. (3)	a-	meno			-rrhea
25. (2)		oo			-cyst
26. (2)		oo			-genic
27. (2)	dys-				-tocia
28. (2)	multi-				-para
29. (2)	primi-				-para
30. (2)		perimetri			-ectomy
31. (2)		pyo			-salpinx
32. (4)		vagino	hystero	toko	-otomy
33. (2)	a-				-tocia
34. (2)		colpo			-sarcoma
35. (3)	dys-	meno			-rrhea

Activity 6

Word Building

1. hysterocervicectomy
2. colpocervicostomy
3. hysterorrhexis
4. oligomenorrhea
5. oo-oophorocentesis
   oooophorocentesis
6. dysmenorrhea
7. hysterosalpingopexy
8. hysterosalpingoptosis
9. hemosalpinx, hematosalpinx
10. salpingohysteroanastomosis
11. trachelomyometriorrhaphy
12. panhysterectomy
13. oo-oophorotomy, oooophorotomy
14. endometriolysis
15. tracheloatresia, trachelatresia
16. myometrioma
17. cervicosarcoma
18. endocervicitis
19. intratrachelotherapy
20. embryology
21. intrauteropyosis
22. colpocervicodynia
23. laparohysterotokotomy
24. genitopathology
25. colpovulvocervicoplasty

Activity 7

Defining Medical Terms

1.	colpo	-pexy		suspension of vagina
2.	colpo	-ptosis		prolapse of vagina
3.	salpingo	oophoro	-plasty	reconstruction of uterine tubes and ovaries
4.	salpingo	-rrhagia		bleeding of the fallopian tubes
5.	salpingo	-rrhexis		rupture of oviduct(s)
6.	salpingo	uter	-ostomy	anastomosis of uterus to oviducts
7.	salpingo	oophor	-pexy	suspension of the salpinges (plural) and ovaries
8.	ovario	-centesis		puncture for aspiration of ovaries (ovary)
9.	oophoro	-centesis		tapping of ovaries (ovary)
10.	colpo	-scope		instrument used to view the vagina
11.	salping	-itis		inflammation of the fallopian tubes
12.	vagin	-itis		inflammation of vagina
13.	salpingo	-ptosis		prolapse of oviducts
14.	cervico	colpo	-plasty	reconstruction of cervix and vagina
15.	salping	-ectomy		excision of fallopian tube(s)
16.	gynec	-ology		study of medical conditions of female
17.	cervic	-algia		pain of cervix
18.	procto	colpo	-cele	herniation of rectum and vagina
19.	a-	meno	-rrhea	no menstruation
20.	trachel	-itis		inflammation of cervix
21.	endo-	vagin	-al	concerning within the vagina (lining of vagina)

Activity 7

Defining Medical Terms (continued)

#					Definition
22.	pan-	hyster	-ectomy		surgical removal of the entire uterus and cervix
23.	intra-	vagin	-al		concerning inside the vagina
24.	salpingo	oophor	-ectomy		surgical removal oviduct(s) and ovaries (ovary)
25.	pan-	oophoro	salpingo	hyster -ectomy	excision of both ovaries, oviducts, uterus and cervix
26.	endometrio	-lysis			freeing up or breakdown of the endometrium
27.	perine	-otomy			incision into the perineum
28.	meno	-rrhea			monthly flow, menstruation
29.	episi	-otomy			incision of perineum and/or vulva
30.	dys-	meno	-rrhea		painful monthly flow, "cramps"
31.	oo	-kinesis			movement of the ovum
32.	a-	-tocia			no labor
33.	dys-	-tocia			difficult labor
34.	neo-	nat	-al		concerning the newborn
35.	vagino	hystero	tok	-otomy	incision into uterus for delivery through vagina; vaginal C-section
36.	multi-	-para			woman who has borne more than one viable fetus
37.	hemi-	myometrio	-plegia		paralysis of half the muscles of the uterus
38.	nulli-	-gravida			a woman who has never been pregnant
39.	pyo	-salpinx			pus in the oviduct(s)
40.	perimetri	-ectomy			excision of the serosa of uterus
41.	colpo	-stenosis			narrowing of the vagina

Activity 7

Defining Medical Terms (continued)

42. oo   -genic   concerning the production of ova
43. primi-   -para   woman who has delivered or is delivering her first living child
44. trachel   -odynia   cervical pain
45. utero   -paresis   weakness of the uterine structure

Activity 8

Word Building from a Sentence

1. excision of   entire   uterus (including the cervix)
   -ectomy   pan-   hystero   panhysterectomy
2. formation of a communication   vagina   cervix
   -ostomy   vagino   cervico   vaginocervicostomy
   or   -anastomosis   colpo   trachelo   colpotracheloanastomosis
3. rupture of   uterus
   -rrhexis   hystero   hysterorrhexis
4. scanty   menstrual   flow
   oligo-   meno   -rrhea   oligomenorrhea
5. breakdown of   endometrium
   -lysis   endometrio   endometriolysis
6. incision into   ovary   ovum
   -otomy   oophoro   oo   oo-oophorotomy, oooophorotomy
                          ovario   oo   oo-ovariotomy, ooovariotomy
7. blood in   fallopian tubes
   hemo, hemato   salpingo   hemosalpinges, hematosalpinges

Activity 8

Word Building from a Sentence (continued)

#					
8.	joining of -ostomy -anastomosis	uterus hystero	salpinges salpingo		 hysteropansalpingostomy hysteropansalpingoanastomosis
9.	sewing of -rrhaphy	the cervix trachelo cervico	uterine muscle myometrio		 trachelomyometriorrhaphy cervicomyometriorrhaphy
10.	prolapse of -ptosis	uterus hystero			 hysteroptosis
11.	puncture for aspiration -centesis	ovary oophoro ovario	ovum oo oo		 oo-oophorocentesis oo-ovariocentesis
12.	painful dys-	menstruation (monthly flow) meno	 -rrhea		 dysmenorrhea
13.	suspension of -pexy	uterus hystero	fallopian tubes salpingo		 hysterosalpingopexy
14.	suturing of -rrhaphy	vagina colpo	labia majora vulvo		 colpovulvorrhaphy
15.	rupture of -rrhexis	lining (within) endo-	oviduct salpingo		 endosalpingorrhexis
16.	reconstruction of -plasty	vagina colpo vagino	vulva vulvo episio	cervix cervico trachelo	 cervicocolpovuloplasty trachelovagino-episioplasty
17.	herniation of -cele	vagina colpo	bladder cysto		 colpocystocele

Activity 8

Word Building from a Sentence (continued)

18.	cervical	cancer			cervicocarcinoma
	cervico	-carcinoma			trachelocarcinoma
	or trachelo				
19.	tumor of	uterine muscle			
	-oma	myometrio			myometrioma
20.	inflammation of	cervical	lining		
	-itis	trachelo	endo-		endotrachelitis
	or	cervico			endocervicitis
21.	abnormal condition of	pus	inside	uterus	
	-osis	pyo	intra-	hystero	intrahysteropyosis
22.	pain in	vagina	cervix		
	-algia	colpo	cervico		colpocervicalgia
	-dynia	vagino	trachelo		vaginotrachelodynia
23.	cutting through	abdominal wall	uterus	deliver a child	
	-otomy	laparo	hystero	toko	laparohysterotokotomy
24.	excision of	entire	uterus	cervix	
	-ectomy		hystero	trachelo	hysterotrachelectomy
	-ectomy	pan-	hystero		panhysterectomy
25.	absence of normal opening	cervix			
	-atresia	cervico			cervicoatresia, cervicatresia

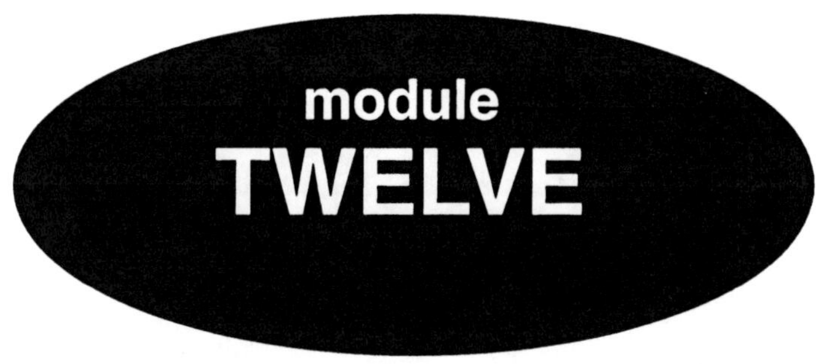

Select Components of the Circulatory, Nervous, Senses and Integumentary Systems

This module contains components frequently seen and used that are related to the system not addressed in other Modules. There are no activities included. See how well you can define words found in your daily reading.

Nervous System

1.	cephalo	head
2.	encephalo	brain
3.	cerebello	cerebellum
4.	cerebro	cerebrum
5.	myelo	spinal cord

Circulatory System and Accessory Components

1.	cardio	heart
2.	myocardio	myocardium: muscle of heart
3.	endocardio	endocardium: lining of heart
4.	pericardio	pericardium: serosa of heart
5.	atrio	atrium (atria, pl.): upper chambers of the heart
6.	auriculo	auricle(s): atrium (atria)
7.	ventriculo	ventricle(s): lower chambers of heart
8.	angio	vessel – general term
9.	hemangio	blood vessel
10.	telangio	capillaries
11.	veno	vein(s)
12.	phlebo	vein(s) – most commonly used
13.	arterio	artery (arteries, pl.)
14.	hemo, hemato	blood
15.	thrombo	thrombus (thrombi, pl.): blood clot fixed to the wall of a bloodvessel
16.	embolo	embolus (emboli, pl.): undisolved foreign matter present in bloodstream
17.	spleno	spleen
18.	lieno	spleen
19.	lympho	lymph
20.	lymphadeno	lymph gland/node
21.	lymphangio	lymph vessel
22.	lymphonodo	lymph node/gland
23.	–angiectasis	distention of a vessel
24.	–stasis	pooling, stagnant

The Sensory and Integumentary System

The Eye

1.	ophthalmo	the eye
2.	oculo	the eye
3.	opto	vision: the ability to see
4.	–opsia, –opia	vision
5.	blepharo	eyelid
6.	palpebro	eyelid
7.	conjunctivo	conjunctiva: mucosa of eye
8.	retino	retina
9.	dacryo	tears
10.	lacrimo	tears
11.	sclero	sclera: white of the eyes

The Ear

1.	oto	ear
2.	auri	ear; ear-shaped
3.	acouso	hearing: the ability to hear
4.	–cusis	hearing
5.	audio, audito	hearing
6.	presby–	old age

The Skin and Related Components

1.	dermo, dermato	skin
2.	tricho	hair
3.	onycho	nails – finger and/or toe
4.	–onychia	nails
5.	mammo, mamma	breast(s)
6.	pachy–	thickening
7.	–geusia	the sense of taste
8.	lepto–	thin, slender

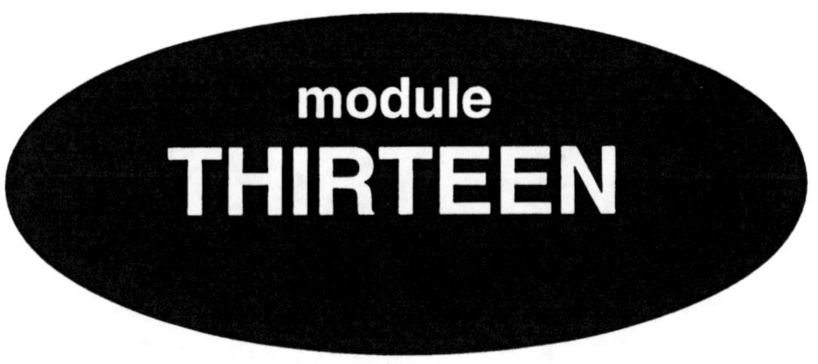

Glossary

A. Suffixes

Suffix	*Meaning of Suffix*
1. –ac, –al, –ar, –ary, –ic	a. pertaining to b. having to do with c. concerning
2. –algia	a. pain
3. –anastomosis	a. a natural or surgical connection of two tubular structures
4. –atresia	a. absence of a normal body opening
5. –carcinoma (carcinoma)*	a. malignant tumor of epithelial tissue b. cancer of epithelial tissue: tissue that lines or covers the body organs or body cavities, skin
6. –cele	a. herniation: abnormal protrusion of an organ or tissue through a defect or any normal internal opening of body
7. –centesis	a. puncture for aspiration b. puncture for removal of any body fluid or air c. tapping for drainage
8. –cision	a. to cut, cutting
9. –clasis	a. surgical refracture
10. –cyst	a. bladder
11. –cyte(s)	a. cell(s)
12. –desis	a. surgical binding (pertains to connective tissue)
13. –dipsia	a. thirst
14. –dynia	a. pain
15. –ectasis –ectasia	a. dilation b. stretching open c. distention
16. –ectomy	a. surgical removal b. excision of c. cutting out
17. –emia	a. present in the bloodstream
18. –emesis (emesis)	a. vomiting b. to vomit
19. –esthesia (esthesia)	a. feeling b. sensation c. perception

Note: ( )* indicate usage of component as a word.

Suffix	*Meaning of Suffix*

20. –genic
    a. originating
    b. origin
    c. producing

21. –gram
    a. a visible or written record or picture (X–ray)
    b. a recorded picture or record (is visible or written)

electro– (root word) –gram
    a. a tracing of electrical activity of a body structure e.g. the muscles or brain

22. –graph
    a. instrument for making a written record, tracing or picture
    b. instrument to record

23. –graphy
    a. process of recording
    b. making a tracing or picture

24. –gravid (gravid)
    a. pregnant, pregnancy

25. –gravida (gravida)
    a. pregnant woman

26. –iasis
    a. presence of (implies presence of foreign matter)
    b. condition of having

27. –ism
    a. characteristic of
    b. having to do with
    c. state of, condition of

28. –itis
    a. inflammation of
    b. inflammatory process: tissues are red, hot, swollen with pain and/or itching

29. –kinesis, –kinesia (kinesis)
    a. movement (muscle), motion

30. –ligation
    a. procedure for tying

31. –lith(s)
    a. stone(s)

32. –lithiasis (lithiasis)
    a. presence of stone(s) in body, presence of calculus (calculi–pl.)

33. –lithotomy (lithotomy)
    a. incision for removal of stone(s)

34. –lysis (lysis)
    a. dissolution, decomposition
    b. breakdown
    c. freeing up, relief of

35. –malacia (malacia)
    a. softening of

36. –megaly / –megalia
    a. enlargement of
    b. large
    c. enlarged

Suffix	*Meaning of Suffix*
37. –natal, –nate (natal)	a. pertaining to birth, birthday
38. –oid	a. resembling b. like
39. –oma	a. tumor (–oma may denote a benign or cancerous tumor)
40. –ology	a. study of
41. –orexia	a. appetite
42. –ostomy (ostomy)	a. more or less permanent opening b. artificial surgical opening c. anastomosis: joining two or more cavities or tubular structures to allow a continuous flow d. joining of two or more tubular structures to allow a continuous flow e. see Module 2.E. "Irregularities"
43. –osis	a. abnormal condition b. increase in condition
44. –osmia, osmo–	a. sense of smell, osmesis
45. –otomy	a. incision into, of, or for b. temporary opening c. cutting into, of or for
46. –ous	a. full of b. abundance of
47. –oxia	a. oxygen (usually in the bloodstream)
48. –para (para)	a. woman having carried a viable (living) fetus beyond the 20th week of pregnancy regardless of whether it was alive at birth
49. –paresis (paresis)	a. weakness
50. –pathy	a. disease
51. –penia	a. deficiency b. decrease c. poverty
52. –pepsia	a. digestion
53. –pexy	a. surgical suspension (pertains to non-epithelial connective tissue or internal organs)
54. –phagia	a. swallowing b. swallow c. eating

Suffix	*Meaning of Suffix*
55. –phasia	a. speech–coherence and comprehension b. speaking words
56. –phonia	a. voice b. vocal sounds c. sounds of speech
57. –plasia –plasm	a. tissue formation (related to number of cells)
58. –plakia	a. patches, plaques
59. –plasty	a. plastic repair b. surgical reconstruction
60. –plegia	a. paralysis: inability to move voluntarily
61. –pnea	a. breathe b. breathing c. breath
62. –poiesis	a. formation of b. manufacturing of
63. –porosis	a. porous b. lessened in density
64. –ptosis –ptosia (ptosis)	a. downward displacement b. prolapse c. drooping d. floating
65. –ptysis (ptysis)	a. spitting b. expectorating
66. –rrhage –rrhagia	a. bleeding b. abnormal flow (usually refers to blood) c. abnormal discharge of blood (rapid discharge)
67. –rrhea	a. flow of any fluid except blood or pus b. discharge (usually not blood)
68. –rrhaphy	a. suture b. surgical repair c. to sew
69. –rrhexis	a. rupture: abrupt separation of tissue
70. –sarcoma (sarcoma)	a. malignant tumor of connective tissue b. cancer of non–epithelial tissue c. malignancy of fleshy tissue
71. –sclerosis (sclerosis)	a. hardening of
72. –scope (scope)	a. instrument used for viewing or examining b. instrument to look through when viewing or examining

Suffix	*Meaning of Suffix*
73. –scopy	a. using an instrument for viewing or examining
74. –spasm (spasm)	a. involuntary contractions b. uncontrolled contractions
75. –stenosis (stenosis)	a. narrowing of
76. –sthenia	a. strength
77. –tasis	a. stretching b. elongation
78. –therapy	a. treatment (therapy)
79. –tocia	a. process of birth, labor
80. –tonos, –tonia	a. muscle tone, muscle elasticity
81. –tripsy	a. crushing (intentionally)
82. –trophy	a. cell nourishment (related to size of cells)
83. –uresis (uresis)	a. urination b. passage of urine c. voiding
84. –ureter	a. ureter(s): one tube from each kidney forming passage for urine to bladder
85. –urethra	a. urethra: tube forming passage of urine from bladder to outside of body
86. –uria	a. present in the urine b. pertaining to urine

B. Prefixes

Prefix	*Meaning of Prefix*
1. a–, (affix to component starting with a consonant) an–, (affix to component starting with a vowel)	a. not b. without c. absent d. absence of
2. ab–	a. away from
3. acro–	a. extremity b. appendage
4. ad–	a. toward, to
5. ante–	a. before
6. anti–	a. against b. opposed
7. atelo–	a. incomplete developmental formation or expansion
8. auto–	a. self
9. bi–	a. two b. twice c. double
10. brady–	a. slow
11. circum–	a. around b. on all sides
12. con– com– (affix to components beginning with b, p, m)	a. with b. together c. in association with
13. contra–	a. against b. opposite
14. crypto–	a. hidden b. a recessed chamber
15. dextro–	a. to the right b. on the right side
16. di–	a. double b. twice c. two
17. dys–	a. bad b. difficult c. painful
18. ecto–	a. outside (normal location) b. external
19. endo–	a. within b. inner

Prefix	*Meaning of Prefix*
20. epi–	a. upon b. over (position)
21. eu–	a. healthy b. normal c. good d. well
22. ex–	a. out of b. from
23. extra–	a. outside of b. in addition to
24. hemi–	a. half (right or left side)
25. homo–	a. same
26. hyper–	a. excessive b. increase c. more than normal d. above
27. hypo–	a. less than b. decrease c. less than normal d. below e. under
28. infra–	a. below (located below another structure)
29. inter–	a. between
30. intra–	a. within b. inside
31. latero–	a. side
32. macro–	a. large
33. micro–	a. small
34. multi–	a. many b. much
35. neo–	a. new b. recent
36. nulli–	a. never b. none
37. oligo–	a. scant b. few c. a little
38. pan–	a. all b. every c. total

Prefix	*Meaning of Prefix*
39. para–	a. near b. beside c. adjacent to d. beyond
40. peri–	a. around b. surrounding
41. poly–	a. many (more than normal) b. much (more than normal)
42. post–	a. behind b. after c. later
43. primi–	a. first b. one
44. pro–	a. before b. in favor of c. forward
45. pseudo–	a. false
46. quadri–	a. four
47. recti–	a. straight
48. retro–	a. behind b. backward
49. semi–	a. half (partial amount) (used in anatomy, rarely in medical terminology)
50. sinistro–	a. to the left b. left side
51. sub–	a. under b. below c. beneath d. in small quantity e. less than normal
52. super–	a. above average b. beyond the normal to an especially high degree
53. supra–	a. above (a location or position)
54. syn– sym– (affixed to components beginning with b, p, m)	a. together
55. tachy–	a. rapid b. fast

Prefix	*Meaning of Prefix*
56. trans–	a. across
	b. over
57. tri–	a. three
58. uni–	a. one

C. Combining Forms

Root Combining Form	*Meaning of Combining Form*
1. abdomino	abdomen
2. albo	white
3. albumino	albumin
4. alveolo	alveolus, sing. (alveoli, pl.): air sacs of the lungs, *parenchyma* of lungs
5. amnio	amniotic fluid, fluid surrounding the fetus
6. andro	man, male
7. ano	anus
8. appendico appendo	appendix – used with any component appendix – form used with –ectomy
9. arthro	joint
10. balano	glans penis
11. bronchio	bronchial tree or tubes of the respiratory system (bronchi and bronchioles)
12. bronchiolo	small branches of respiratory tree; bronchioles
13. broncho	large branches of respiratory tree bronchus – sing., bronchi – pl.
14. bucco	cheeks
15. burso	bursa (bursae–pl.)
16. calco, calcio	calcium
17. carpo	wrist (bones of)
18. ceco	cecum
19. cephalo	head
20. cervico trachelo	uterine cervix, the neck of the uterus; both components may refer to the part of the body connecting the head and the trunk or to the uterine cervix.
21. cheilo	oral lips
22. chloro	green
23. chole	bile, gall
24. cholangio	hepatic duct
25. cholecysto	gallbladder; cholecyst
26. choledocho	common bile duct
27. chondro	cartilage: gristle
28. chromo chromato	color

Root Combining Form	*Meaning of Combining Form*
29. claviculo cleido	clavicle: collar bone
30. colo colono	colon (large intestine)
31. colpo vagino	vagina
32. costo	ribs
33. cranio	cranium: skull
34. cyano	blue
35. cysto	urinary bladder, bladder: a fluid–filled sac containing any fluid except blood or pus
36. dactylo	fingers/toes, digits
37. dento	teeth
38. diaphysio diaphyseo	diaphysis: shaft of long bone
39. duodeno	duodenum: first part of small intestine
40. endometrio	endometrium: lining of the uterus, mucosa of the uterus
41. endosteo	endosteum: lining of the bone
42. entero	intestines, general component for all intestines, both small and large
43. epididymo	epididymis
44. epiphysio epiphyseo	epiphysis: growth end of long bone
45. episio	the perineum and/or the vulva
46. erythro	red
47. esophago	esophagus
48. fascio	fascia: connective tissue that covers muscle
49. femoro	femur: thigh bone
50. feto	fetus
51. fibulo	fibula: small bone of lower leg
52. gastro	stomach
53. genito	reproductive organs
54. gingivo	gingiva: gums
55. glosso, –glossia	tongue
56. gluco	sugar

Root Combining Form	*Meaning of Combining Form*
57. glyco, glycoso	sugar, sweet
58. gyneco gyne gyno	woman, women
59. hemo, hemato	blood
60. hepatico hepato	liver
61. humero	humerus: bone of upper arm
62. hydro	fluid: any body fluid except blood or pus
63. hystero	uterus
64. ileo	ileum: third part of small intestine
65. jejuno	jejunum: second part of small intestine
66. labio	labia, any lip–like structure
67. laparo	abdominal wall: flank
68. laryngo	larynx: voicebox, vocal cords
69. leiomyo	smooth muscle: involuntary muscles, muscles of the *viscera*
70. leuko leuco	white
71. ligamento	ligament: connective tissue which connects bone to bone. This form usually used for anatomical descriptions.
72. lipo lipido	fat
73. litho, –lith(s),	stone(s), calculus (calculi, pl.)
74. lobo	lobes of an organ
75. meato	meatus: opening or passage
76. mediastino	mediastinum: cavity between lungs containing the heart, its large vessels and the esophagus
77. melano	black
78. meno	menstruation, menses (literally, monthly)
79. metro, metrio –metrium (noun suffix)	uterus, usually refers to the uterine muscular structure
80. myelo	bone marrow; spinal cord
81. myo myoso	muscle: meat of body

Root Combining Form	*Meaning of Combining Form*
82. myometrio	myometrium: muscle of the uterus
83. naso	nose
84. nasopharyngo	intracranial passage connecting the nose to the throat
85. nephro	kidney
86. oo	ovum (ova, pl.), egg(s)
87. oophoro ovario	ovary (ovaries, pl.)
88. orchio orchido	testis, sing. (testes, pl.), testicle(s)
89. oro, ora	mouth, used to indicate the anatomical structure or pertaining to; not commonly used in forming medical words
90. osteo	bone
91. palato	hard palate (roof of the mouth)
92. pancreato pancreatico	pancreas
93. pedo pedio	child (children)
94. pelvo pelvi pelvio	pelvis, pelvic cavity
95. peno phallo	penis
96. perimetrio	perimetrium: serosa of the uterus, tissue covering the outside of the uterus
97. perineo	perineum: the tissue forming the floor of the pelvic cavity located between the vulva and the rectum in both the male and female
98. periosteo	periosteum: membrane covering bone
99. peritoneo	peritoneum: tissue which forms the serosa of the abdominal cavity
100. phalango	finger(s) and/or toe(s): bones of finger(s)/toe(s)
101. pharyngo	pharynx (throat)
102. pleuro –pleura (noun suffix)	serosa of thorax: pleural membranes pleural cavity, (pleura, sing.), (pleurae, pl.) pleural fluid
103. pneumo	air: used with noun suffix lung: used with regular suffix

Root Combining Form	*Meaning of Combining Form*
104. pneumono, –pneumonon (noun suffix)	lung(s)
105. polio	gray
106. prepuco	prepuce: foreskin
107. procto	rectum and/or anus
108. prostato	prostate gland
109. proteino	protein
110. pulmo pulmono, –pulmonon (noun suffix)	lung(s)
111. pyelo	pelvis (renal)
112. pyo	pus
113. rachio	spinal column: backbone
114. radio	radius: large long bone on thumb side of the forearm
115. recto	rectum
116. reno	kidney (form rarely used in medical terminology)
117. rhabdomyo	striated muscle: voluntary muscle, skeletal muscle
118. rhino	nose
119. rube rubri	red
120. salpingo –salpinx (noun suffix)	salpinx (salpinges, pl.): also called uterine tubes, fallopian tubes, oviducts
121. scroto	scrotum
122. sialadeno	salivary gland
123. sialangio	salivary duct
124. sialo	saliva
125. sigmoido	sigmoid colon
126. sinuso	sinus
127. spermatozoo spermato	spermatozoon, sing. (spermatoza, pl.): mature male sex cell
128. spino	spine: any bony projection
129. spondylo	vertebra, (vertebrae–pl): individual bones of spinal column
130. stomato	mouth, refers to oral mouth only

Root Combining Form	*Meaning of Combining Form*
131. syndesmo	ligament: component usually used in medical terminology
132. synovio	synovial membrane/fluid
133. tendino tendo tendono teno	tendon: connective tissue which connects bone to muscle
134. testo testiculo	testicle(s)
135. thoraco thora (rare variation)	chest, chest cavity, thorax chest (used with –centesis only)
136. tibio	tibia: shin bone of lower leg
137. toco, toko	birth, process of birth
138. tonsillo	tonsil(s)
139. tracheo	trachea: windpipe
140. ulno	ulna: smaller long bone on the little finger side of the forearm
141. ureter	ureter(s)
142. urethro	urethra
143. uro	urinary system, urinary tract, urine
144. utero	uterus, usually use as an anatomical reference
145. vaso	inclusive component for sperm carrying tubular structures: vas deferens, ejaculatory duct and seminal duct
146. vertebro	vertebra: individual bones of the spinal column. Used in anatomy, not used for medical terms
147. viri	male, masculine
148. viscero	viscera, pl. (visceus, sing.): internal organ enclosed within a cavity
149. vulvo	vulva; in anatomy: labia majora
150. xantho	yellow

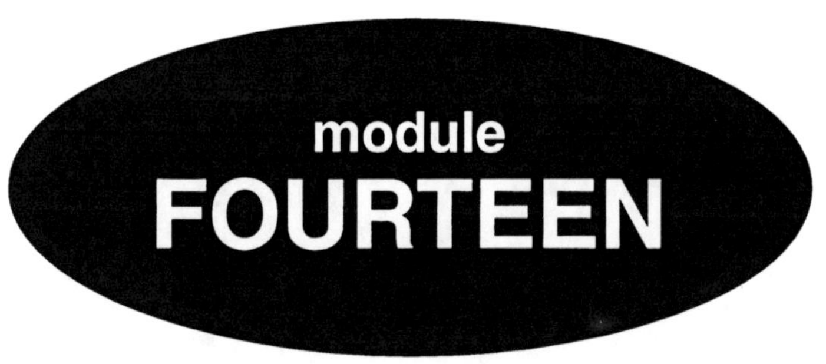

Medical Terminology Abbreviations

Medical Terminology Abbreviations

Common Prescription Abbreviations and Symbols

a	before
ac	before meals
amt	amount
bid	twice a day
$\bar{c}$	with
cap(s)	capsule
dil	dilute
D_5W	5% dextrose in water
gt; gtt	drop; drops
H or hr	hour
hs	at bedtime
IM	intramuscular
IV	intravenous
NS	normal saline
oint	ointment
oz	ounce
p	after
per	by or with
pc	after meals
po	by mouth
prn	when necessary
q	every
qd	every day
qh	every hour
q_h	every___hour (example: q2h – every 2 hours)
qid	four times a day
qod	every other day
qns	quantity not sufficient
Rx	prescription, (take thou)
$\bar{s}$	without
sc or subq	subcutaneous
Sig	let it be labeled
ss or $\bar{\bar{ss}}$	one-half

subling	sublingual (under the tongue)
tid	three times a day
tab	tablet
TPN	total parenteral nutrition
ung	ointment

Metric — use no periods or upper case letters except L

cc	cubic centimeter
gm	gram
kg	kilogram
L	liter
mg	milligram
ml	milliliter
mm	millimeter

Body systems

HEENT	head, eyes, ear, nose and throat
CR	cardiorespiratory
CVS	cardiovascular
GI	gastrointestinal
GU	genito-urinary
CNS	central nervous system
MS	musculo-skeletal
NM	neuro-muscular

Patient's History

CC	chief complaint
c/o	complains of
DOB	date of birth
H & P	history and physical
PI or HPI	(history of) present illness
FH	family history
PH	past history
UCHD or UCD	usual childhood diseases
a & w	alive and well
PTA	prior to admission
LMD	local medical doctor

Physical Exam

ax	axillary
wd	well developed
wn	well nourished
P & A	percussion and auscultation
BP	blood pressure
TPR	temperature, pulse, respiration
VS	vital signs
WNL	within normal limits
wt	weight
ht	height

Diagnosis

Dx	diagnosis
R/O	rule out
Bx	biopsy
NIDDM	non-insulin-dependent diabetes mellitus
IDDM	insulin-dependent diabetes mellitus

Eye

REM	rapid eye movement
OS	left eye
OD	right eye
OU	both eyes

Chest (heart and lung)

SOB	short of breath
NSR	normal sinus rhythm
MI	myocardial infarction
EKG or ECG	electrocardiogram
CHF	congestive heart failure
COPD	chronic obstructive pulmonary disease
CAD	coronary artery disease
CABG	coronary artery bypass graft

Abdomen and GI

abd	abdomen
GB	gallbladder
BM	bowel movement

Female

D&C	dilatation and curettage
LMP	last menstrual period
OB	obstetrics
PID	pelvic inflammatory disease
GYN	gynecology
EDC	expected date of confinement
L & D	labor and delivery
PP	postpartum

Male

| BPH | benign prostatic hypertrophy |
| TURP | transurethral resection of prostate |

Musculoskeletal

DTR	deep tendon reflexes
Fx	fracture
ROM	range of motion

Central Nervous System

| CSF | cerebral spinal fluid |
| CVA | cerebrovascular accident |

General

Ca or CA	cancer
d/c or D/C	discontinue
DOA	dead on arrival or date of admission
OD	overdose
stat	immediately
ad lib	as desired
BR	bed rest
I & O	intake and output

LP	lumbar puncture
FUO	fever of unknown origin
GC	gonococcus (gonorrhea)
PM	post mortem
PAT	pre admission testing
pt	patient
Lt	left
Rt	right
BRP	bathroom privileges
CXR	chest x-ray
GSW	gunshot wound
lytes	electrolytes
NKA	no known allergies
NPO	nothing by mouth
VO	verbal orders
TO	telephone orders
DNR	do not resuscitate
AIDS	acquired immune deficiency syndrome
HIV	human immuno-deficiency virus
♂	male
♀	female

Laboratory

CBC	complete blood count
HGB or HG or Hb	hemoglobin
Hct or hct	hematocrit
WBC	white blood count (white blood cell)
RBC	red blood count (red blood cell)
FBS	fasting blood sugar
C & S	culture and sensitivity
ABG	arterial blood gases

Departments

ICU	intensive care unit
CCU	coronary care unit
ER	emergency room

OR	operating room
RR or PAR	recovery room or postanesthetic room
Lab	laboratory
Path	pathology
OPD	outpatient department
Peds	pediatrics
RT	respiratory therapy
PT	physical therapy
STAT, stat	immediately
ASAP	as soon as possible